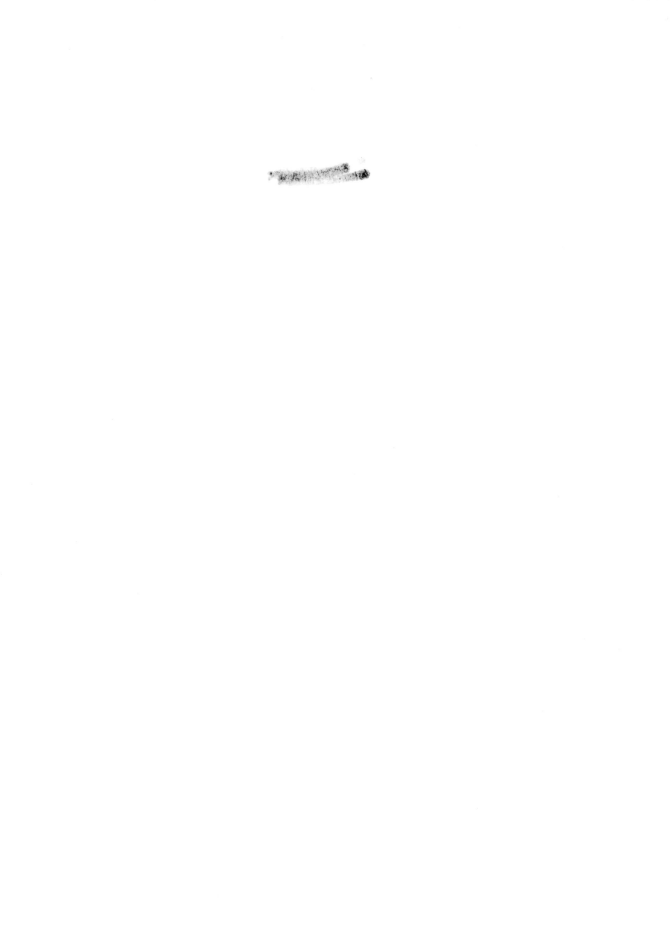

Atlas of the
Newborn

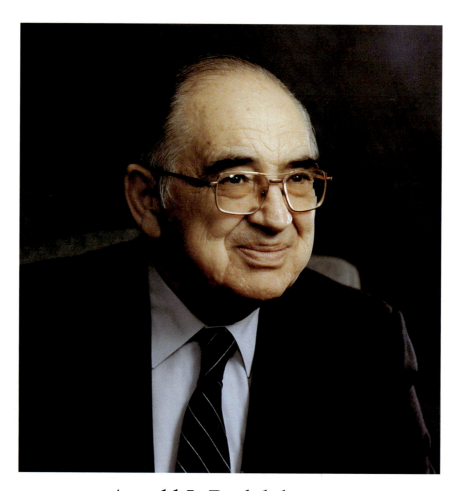

Arnold J. Rudolph, M.D.
1918–1995
Professor of Pediatrics,
Obstetrics and Gynecology
Baylor College of Medicine
Houston, Texas

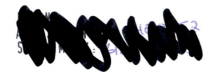

VOLUME 4

Dermatology and Perinatal Infection

Atlas of the Newborn

Arnold J. Rudolph, M.D.
1918–1995

1997

B.C. Decker Inc.
Hamilton • London

B.C. Decker Inc.
4 Hughson Street South
P.O. Box 620, L.C.D. 1
Hamilton, Ontario L8N 3K7
Tel: 905 522-7017
Fax: 905 522-7839
e-mail: info@bcdecker.com

Printed in Canada

97 98 99 00/BP/9 8 7 6 5 4 3 2 1

ISBN 1-55009-034-8

Sales and distribution

United States
Blackwell Science Inc.
Commerce Place
350 Main Street
Malden, MA 02148
U.S.A.
Tel: 1-800-215-1000

Canada
Copp Clark Ltd.
200 Adelaide Street West
3rd Floor
Toronto, Ontario
Canada M5H 1W7
Tel: 416-597-1616
Fax: 416-597-1617

Japan
Igaku-Shoin Ltd.
Tokyo International P.O. Box 5063
1-28-36 Hongo, Bunkyo-ku
Tokyo 113, Japan
Tel: 3 3817 5680
Fax: 3 3815 7805

U.K., Europe, Scandinavia, Middle East
Blackwell Science Ltd.
c/o Marston Book Services Ltd.
P.O. Box 87
Oxford OX2 0DT
England
Tel: 44-1865-79115

Australia
Blackwell Science Pty, Ltd.
54 University Street
Carleton, Victoria 3053
Australia
Tel: 03 9347 0300
Fax: 03 9349 3016

Foreword

Sir William Osler stated, "There is no more difficult task in medicine than the art of observation." The late Arnold Jack Rudolph was an internationally renowned neonatologist, a teacher's teacher, and, above all, one who constantly reminded us about how much could be learned by simply observing, in his case, the newborn infant.

This color atlas of neonatology represents a distillation of more than 50 years of observing normal and abnormal newborn infants. The *Atlas* begins with a section on the placenta, its membranes, and the umbilical cord. Jack Rudolph delighted in giving a lecture entitled "Don't Make Mirth of the Afterbirth," in which he captivated audiences by showing them how much you could learn about the newborn infant from simply observing the placenta, its membranes, and the umbilical cord.

In a few more than 60 photomicrographs, we learn to read the placenta and gain insight into such disorders as intrauterine growth retardation, omphalitis, cytomegalic inclusion disease, congenital syphilis, and congenital neuroblastoma. Congenital abnormalities of every organ system are depicted along with the appearance of newborn infants who have been subjected in utero to a variety of different drugs, toxins, or chemicals. We also learn to appreciate the manifestations of birth trauma and abnormalities caused by abnormal intrauterine positioning.

More than 250 photographs are used to illustrate the field of neonatal dermatology. The collection of photographs used in this section is superior to that which I have seen in any other textbook or atlas of neonatology or dermatology; this section alone makes this reference a required addition to the library of any clinician interested in the care of infants and children. Photographs of the Kasabach-Merritt syndrome (cavernous hemangioma with thrombocytopenia), Klippel-Trenaunay syndrome, Turner's syndrome, Waardenburg's syndrome, neurocutaneous melanosis, mastocytosis (urticaria pigmentosa), and incon-tinentia pigmenti (Bloch-Sulzberger syndrome) are among the best that I have seen.

Cutaneous manifestations are associated with many perinatal infections. The varied manifestations of staphylococcal infection of the newborn are depicted vividly in photomicrographs of furunculosis, pyoderma, bullous impetigo, abscesses, parotitis, dacryocystitis, inastitis, cellulitis, omphalitis, and funisitis. Streptococcal cellulitis, *Haemophilus influenzae* cellulitis, and cutaneous manifestations of listeriosis all are depicted. There are numerous photomicrographs of congenital syphilis, showing the typical peripheral desquamative rash on the palms and soles, as well as other potential skin manifestations of congenital syphilis which may produce either vesicular, bullous, or ulcerative lesions. The various radiologic manifestations of congenital syphilis, including pneumonia alba, ascites, growth arrest lines, Wegner's sign, periostitis, and syphilitic osteochondritis, are depicted. Periostitis of the clavicle (Higouménaki's sign) is shown in a photograph that also depicts periostitis of the ribs. A beautiful photomicrograph of Wimberger's sign also has been included; this sign, which may appear in an infant with congenital syphilis, reveals radiolucency due to erosion of the medial aspect of the proximal tibial metaphysis.

The *Atlas* also includes a beautiful set of photographs which delineate the ophthalmologic examination of the newborn. Lesions which may result from trauma, infection, or congenital abnormalities are included. There are numerous photographs of the ocular manifestations of a variety of systemic diseases, such as Tay-Sachs disease, tuberous sclerosis, tyrosinase deficiency, and many more. Photographs of disturbances of each of the various organ systems, or disorders affecting such organ systems, also are included along with numerous photographs of different forms of dwarfism, nonchromosomal syndromes and associations, and chromosomal disorders. In short, this *Atlas* is the complete visual textbook of neonatology and will provide any physician, nurse, or student with a distillation of 50 years of neonatal experience as viewed through the eyes of a master clinician.

Arnold Jack Rudolph was born in 1918, grew up in South Africa, and graduated from the Witwatersrand Medical School in 1940. Following residency training in pediatrics at the Transvaal Memorial Hospital for Children, he entered private pediatric practice in Johannesburg, South Africa. After almost a decade, he left South Africa and moved to Boston, where he served as a Senior Assistant Resident in Medicine at the Children's Medical Center in Boston, Massachusetts, and subsequently pursued fellowship training in neonatology at the same institution and at the Boston Lying-In Hospital, Children's Medical Center and Harvard Medical School under Dr. Clement A. Smith.

In 1961, Dr. Rudolph came to Baylor College of Medicine in Houston, Texas, the school at which he spent the remainder of his career. He was a master teacher, who received the outstanding teacher award from pediatric medical students on so many occasions that he was elected to the Outstanding Faculty Hall of Fame in 1982. Dr. Rudolph also received numerous awards over the years from the pediatric house staffs for his superb teaching skills.

He was the Director of the Newborn Section in the Department of Pediatrics at Baylor College of Medicine for many years, until he voluntarily relinquished that position in 1986 for reasons related to his health.

Nevertheless, Jack Rudolph continued to work extraordinarily long hours in the care of the newborn infant, and was at the bedside teaching both students and house staff, as well as his colleagues, on a daily basis until just a few months before his death in July 1995.

Although Dr. Rudolph was the author or co-author of more than 100 published papers that appeared in the peer-reviewed medical literature, his most lasting contribution to neonatology and to pediatrics is in the legacy of the numerous medical students, house staff, fellows, and other colleagues whom he taught incessantly about how much one could learn from simply observing the newborn infant. This *Atlas* is a tour de force; it is a spectacular teaching tool that has been developed, collated, and presented by one of the finest clinical neonatologists in the history of medicine. It is an intensely personal volume that, as Dr. Rudolph himself states, "is not intended to rival standard neonatology texts," but rather to supplement them. This statement reveals Dr. Rudolph's innate modesty, since with the exception of some discussion on pathogenesis and treatment, it surpasses most neonatology texts in the wealth of clinical information that one can derive from viewing and imbibing its contents. We owe Dr. Rudolph and those who aided him in this work a debt of gratitude for making available to the medical community an unparalleled visual reference on the normal and abnormal newborn infant.

Ralph D. Feigin, M.D.
June 13, 1996

Preface

I first became attracted to the idea of producing a color atlas of neonatology many years ago. However, the impetus to synthesize my experience and compile this current collection was inspired by the frequent requests from medical students, pediatric house staff, nurses and others to provide them with a color atlas of the clinical material provided in my "slide shows." For the past few decades I have used the medium of color slides and radiographs as a teaching tool. In these weekly "slide shows" the normal and abnormal, as words never can, are illustrated.

"I cannot define an elephant but I know one when I see one."[1]

The collection of material used has been added to constantly with the support of the pediatric house staff who inform me to "bring your camera" whenever they see an unusual clinical finding or syndrome in the nurseries.

A thorough routine neonatal examination is the inalienable right of every infant. Most newborn babies are healthy and only a relatively small number may require special care. It is important to have the ability to distinguish normal variations and minor findings from the subtle early signs of problems. The theme that recurs most often is that careful clinical assessment, in the traditional sense, is the prerequisite and the essential foundation for understanding the disorders of the newborn. It requires familiarity with the wide range of normal, as well as dermatologic, cardiac, pulmonary, gastrointestinal, genitourinary, neurologic, and musculoskeletal disorders, genetics and syndromes. A background in general pediatrics and a working knowledge of obstetrics are essential. The general layout of the atlas is based on the above. Diseases are assigned to each section on the basis of the most frequent and obvious presenting sign. It seems probable that the findings depicted will change significantly in the decades to come. In this way duplication has been kept to a minimum. Additional space has been devoted to those areas of neonatal pathology (e.g., examination of the placenta, multiple births and iatrogenesis) which pose particular problems or cause clinical concern.

Obviously, because of limitations of space, it is impossible to be comprehensive and include every rare disorder or syndrome. I have tried to select both typical findings and variations in normal infants and those found in uncommon conditions. Some relevant conditions where individual variations need to be demonstrated are shown in more than one case.

As the present volume is essentially one of my personal experience, it is not intended to rival standard neonatology texts, but is presented as a supplement to them. It seems logical that references should be to standard texts or reviews where discussion on pathogenesis, treatment, and references to original works may be found.

Helen Mintz Hittner, M.D., has been kind enough to contribute the outstanding section on neonatal ophthalmology.

I have done my best to make the necessary acknowledgements to the various sources for the clinical material. If I have inadvertently omitted any of those, I apologize. My most sincere appreciation and thanks to Donna Hamburg, M.D., Kru Ferry, M.D., Michael Gomez, M.D., Virginia Schneider, PA, and Jeff Murray, M.D., who have spent innumerable hours in organizing and culling the material from my large collection. We wish to thank Abraham M. Rudolph, M.D., for his assistance in reviewing the material. We also wish to thank the following people for their photographic contributions to this work: Gerardo Cabrera-Meza, Morven Edwards, John Kenny, Claire Langston, Moise Levy, Ken Moise and Don Singer.

It is hoped that this atlas will provide neonatologists, pediatricians, family physicians, medical students and nurses with a basis for recognizing a broad spectrum of normal variations and clinical problems as well as provide them with an overall perspective of neonatology, a field in which there continues to be a rapid acceleration of knowledge and technology. One must bear in mind the caveat that pictures cannot supplant clinical experience in mastering the skill of visual recall.

1. Senile dementia of Alzheimer's type — normal aging or disease? (Editorial) *Lancet* 1989; i:476-477.

Arnold J. Rudolph, M.D.

CONTENTS

Volume 4
Dermatology and Perinatal Infection

Introduction

Although several texts provide extensive written descriptions of the newborn infant, the senses of touch, hearing, and especially sight, create the most lasting impressions. Over a period of almost five decades, my brother Jack Rudolph diligently recorded, in pictorial form, his vast experiences in physical examination of the newborn infant. *Atlas of the Newborn* reflects his selection from the thousands of color slides in his collection, and truly represents the "art of medicine" as applied to neonatology. A number of unusual or rare conditions are included in this atlas. I consider this fully justified, because if one has not seen or heard of a condition, one will never be able to diagnose it.

This fourth volume of the five-volume series reviews two main areas; disorders of the skin, and perinatal infections.

Clinical assessment of skin disorders in the newborn infant is one of the most challenging problems confronting neonatologists and pediatricians, and many feel quite insecure in evaluating skin lesions in neonates. Chapter 1, *Dermatology*, provides a unique and elegant collection of color photographs illustrating many of the skin abnormalities that may be encountered in the newborn. The section depicting benign and transient skin lesions is of particular interest, and congenital abnormalities, vascular malformations, disorders of pigmentation, vesiculo-bullous lesions, and scaling conditions are extensively reviewed. This is perhaps the most detailed graphic presentation of dermatologic problems in the newborn infant currently available.

Chapter 2, *Perinatal Infection*, provides excellent illustrations of various organ system involvements in the neonate resulting from infection by bacteria and by syphilis, as well as prenatal viral infections such as cytomegalovirus, rubella, and varicella, and infection by protozoa such as toxoplasma. The section depicting congenital syphilis is especially comprehensive, covering the protean manifestations of this infection in the infant. The effects of neonatally-acquired infections due to bacteria, herpes virus and fungi are also elegantly illustrated.

Volume IV of *Atlas of the Newborn* will be of enormous value to general pediatricians, neonatologists, obstetricians and nurses involved in perinatal care, and also to dermatologists and infectious disease specialists.

Abraham M. Rudolph, M.D.

Chapter 1
Neonatal Dermatology

The neonatal skin must be given careful consideration for several reasons:

- It is a protective organ, especially when covered with vernix.
- Any break in integrity creates an opportunity for infection; therefore, minimize skin trauma.
- Absorption of agents through the skin, especially in premature infants, may have harmful effects (e.g., hexachlorophene, Betadine™, boric acid, etc.)
- The skin may be used therapeutically (e.g., application of safflower oil for essential fatty acid deficiency).

Neonatal skin may present a bewildering variety of lesions; some innocent, temporary and the result of a physiologic response; others the result of an episodic disease; and still others indicative of a serious, often fatal, underlying disorder.

Dermatologic manifestations of infection are presented in Chapter 2, Perinatal Infection.

BENIGN AND TRANSIENT CUTANEOUS LESIONS

These lesions are commonly observed in a normal nursery population, and none require special therapeutic consideration. Numerous benign minor variations in the skin noted in the routine care of babies who are well include skin pigmentation, desquamation, vernix caseosa, etc.

1.1

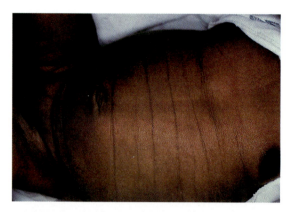

Figure 1.1. In this infant there is a regular segment-like pattern of transverse folding creases across the lower thorax and abdomen giving the trunk a "gridiron" appearance. Note the prominent linea nigra. This finding is more common in postmature infants.

1.2

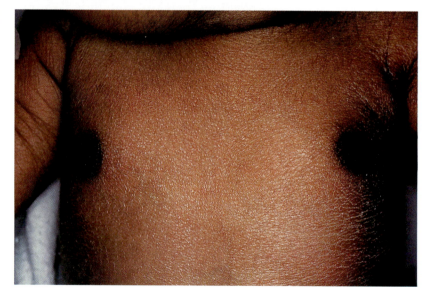

Figure 1.2. Pigmentation of the areola of the nipple in a newborn infant. Pigmentation is more marked in black infants.

1.3

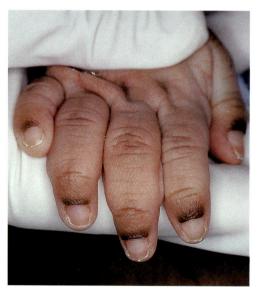

Figure 1.3. Pigmentation at the base of the nails in a black infant. There may be little pigmentation of the skin in general at birth, but the finding of pigmentation at the base of the nails, pinnae of the ears, axilla, areolae of the nipples, genitalia, and a prominent linea nigra would all suggest that the infant is a black infant.

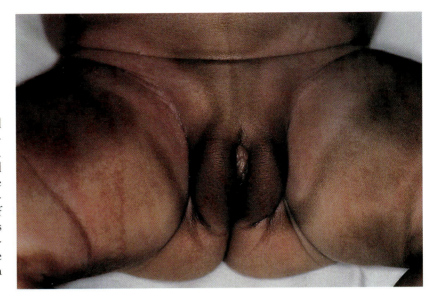

1.4

Figure 1.4. Linea nigra and pigmentation of the skin and genitalia in a black female infant. Linea nigra is the line of increased pigmentation extending from the umbilicus to the more darkly pigmented genitalia. This area of benign pigmentation becomes less prominent as the baby's skin darkens. In this postmature infant note the area of lack of pigmentation in both groins.

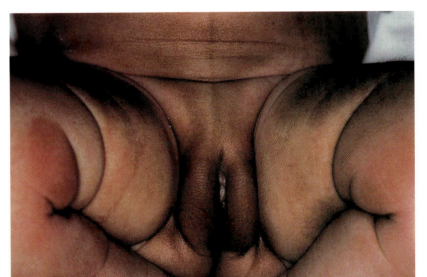

1.5

Figure 1.5. The same infant as in Figure 1.4 with her thighs adducted. Note that the areas lacking pigmentation in the groins correspond to the area protected in utero by adduction of the lower limbs.

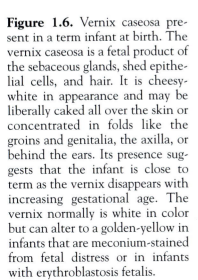

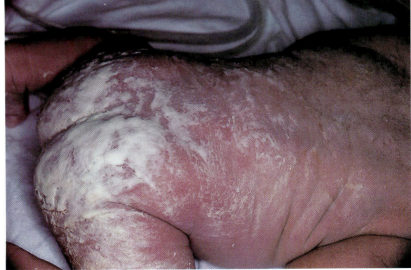

1.6

Figure 1.6. Vernix caseosa present in a term infant at birth. The vernix caseosa is a fetal product of the sebaceous glands, shed epithelial cells, and hair. It is cheesy-white in appearance and may be liberally caked all over the skin or concentrated in folds like the groins and genitalia, the axilla, or behind the ears. Its presence suggests that the infant is close to term as the vernix disappears with increasing gestational age. The vernix normally is white in color but can alter to a golden-yellow in infants that are meconium-stained from fetal distress or in infants with erythroblastosis fetalis.

1.7

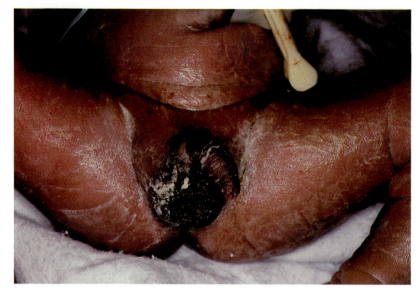

Figure 1.7. A minimal amount of vernix caseosa in the groins and genitalia of a male infant.

1.8

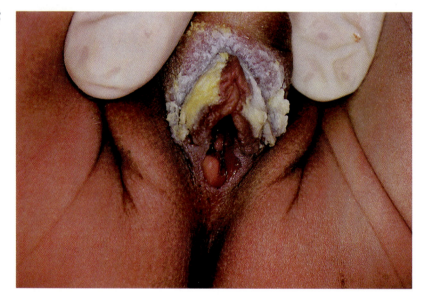

Figure 1.8. Vernix caseosa in a female infant. After birth the infant is bathed and the vernix removed by the nurse. If there is any question as to whether or not there was any meconium staining, certain areas such as the axilla, inguinal folds and genitalia, if not adequately cleaned, will reveal traces of the vernix.

1.9

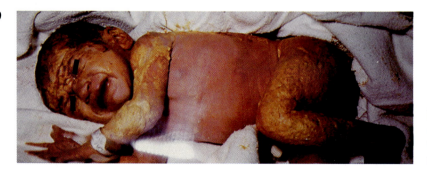

Figure 1.9. Meconium staining of the vernix and skin in an infant who had fetal distress with meconium-stained amniotic fluid.

1.10

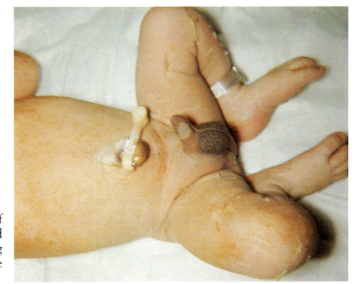

Figure 1.10. Note the meconium staining of the skin in a post-term infant. He also had marked desquamation of the skin as well as long finger nails, features common to the postmature infant.

1.11

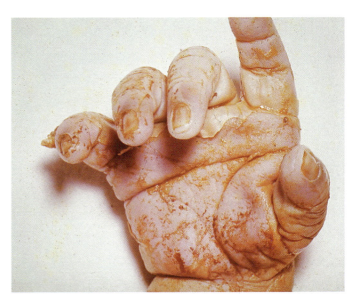

Figure 1.11. The hand of the same infant as in Figure 1.10 showing the desquamation of the skin, long finger nails, and meconium staining.

1.12

Figure 1.12. Marked desquamation of the skin in a post-term infant. This is a benign physiologic desquamation with paper-thin peeling; the underlying skin is normal. It occurs with postmaturity as the vernix disappears and the skin of the fetus is not protected from the amniotic fluid. The process is more marked in areas of irritation.

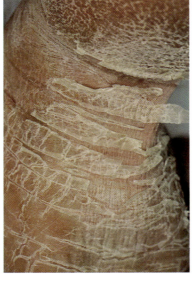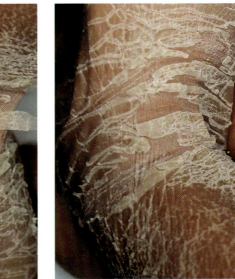

1.13

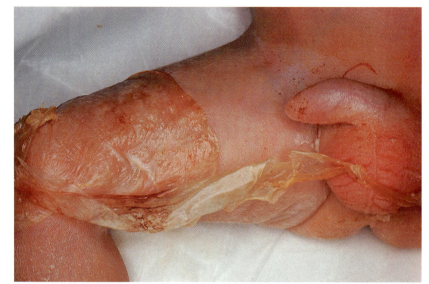

Figure 1.13. Desquamation of the skin is a very typical finding in an abdominal pregnancy in which the fetus is not protected by the amniotic fluid.

1.14

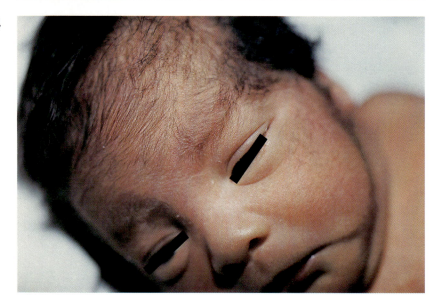

Figure 1.14. Hypertrichosis (hirsutism) is very common in normal mature Hispanic infants.

1.15

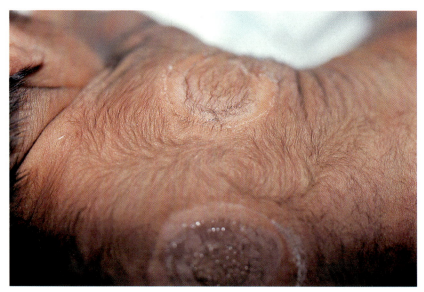

Figure 1.15. Another infant with hypertrichosis over the body at birth. Note that although this is very striking it is a normal finding in normal mature Hispanic infants.

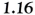

1.16

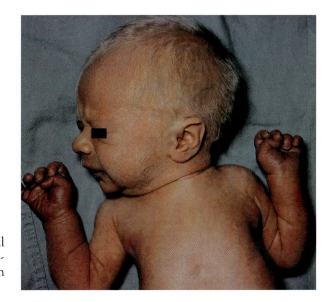

Figure 1.16. Acrocyanosis in an otherwise normal infant. Peripheral vasoconstriction occurs very commonly in normal infants and rapidly improves when the infant is warmed or cries.

1.17

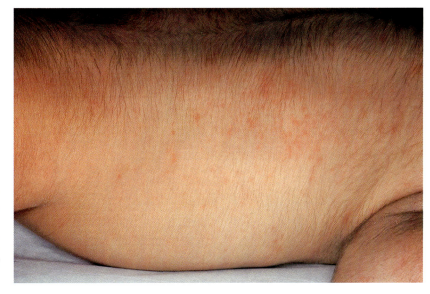

Figure 1.17. In this infant note the maculopapular rash which followed phototherapy treatment for hyperbilirubinemia. This "bilirubin rash" improves rapidly following discontinuation of phototherapy.

1.18

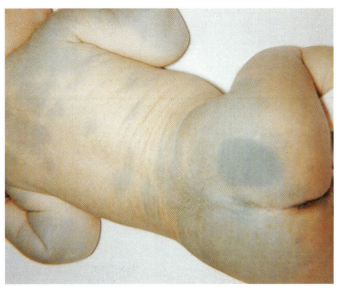

Figure 1.18. Mongolian spots in a caucasian infant. Mongolian spots are a minor anomaly commonly found in infants of darkly pigmented racial groups. They occur in 5 to 10% of caucasian infants, 70% of hispanic and oriental infants, and over 90% of black infants. The circumscribed bluish-grey to dark blue areas of discoloration are usually found over the lumbosacral area and lower back, rarely extending as far as the shoulders and neck, and can also be found on the limbs. They tend to be on the outer surfaces of the body when the infant is placed in its fetal position and are due to an accumulation of dopa-positive melanocytes.

1.19

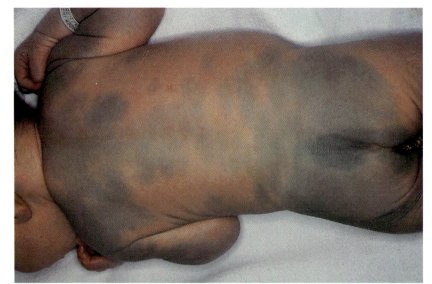

Figure 1.19. Mongolian spots in a black infant. The spots have no significance but are sometimes mistaken for bruises, causing a suspicion of child abuse. This should be kept in mind when intentional injury is questioned. They fade during childhood or appear to fade as the skin darkens. As mongolian spots are never elevated and are not palpable, they can be differentiated from a blue nevus which is raised and is located on the arms, legs, or face and persists throughout life.

1.20

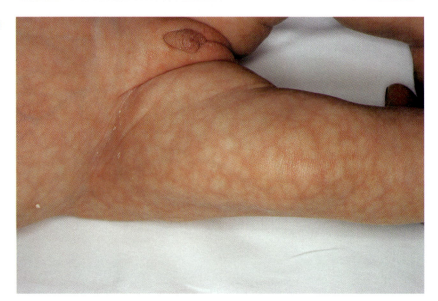

Figure 1.20. Cutis marmorata is a common finding in normal infants. This fine reticulated mottled appearance is due to vasomotor instability and thus is more commonly seen in premature infants, but should also alert one to the possibility of sepsis, hypothyroidism, and central nervous system pathology.

1.21

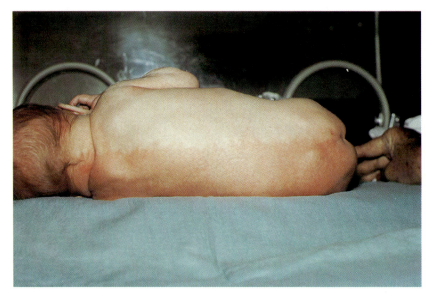

Figure 1.21. In the harlequin sign (harlequin color change) there is a vivid line of demarcation which appears down the midline. The dependent side of the skin becomes flushed (erythematous) and the uppermost side becomes pale. If the infant is turned to the other side, the appearance of the skin reverses. It is proposed that this condition results from vasomotor instability.

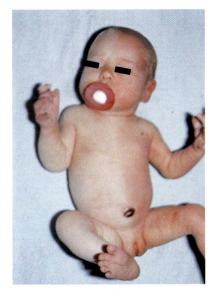
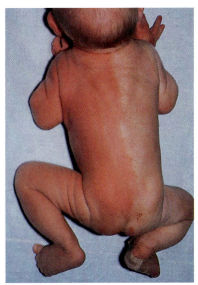

1.22

Figure 1.22. The harlequin sign in another infant showing the frontal and posterior views. This condition occurs most commonly in premature infants, is rare in term infants, and is of no pathologic significance. It may recur repeatedly in the same infant but disappears within the first few months of life. Harlequin sign is not to be confused with the harlequin fetus (ichthyosis congenita).

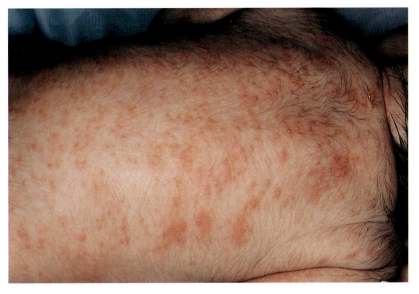

1.23

Figure 1.23. Erythema toxicum neonatorum (urticaria neonatorum) on the back of a term infant. This is the most common rash noted in the normal term infant. It is not seen in preterm and rarely seen in post-term infants. It usually appears on the 2nd or 3rd day of life (rarely in the first 24 hours) and is seldom seen after the age of 14 days. It affects about 40 to 50% of full term infants and the condition is self-limiting. Lesions may be minimal or extensive.

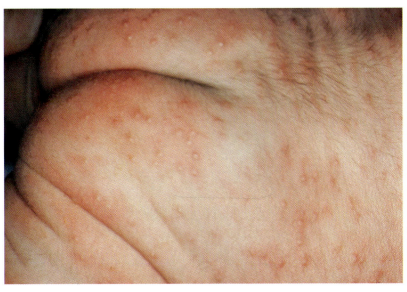

1.24

Figure 1.24. Another example of erythema toxicum neonatorum ("flea bite" dermatitis of the newborn). The lesions most frequently present are erythematous and maculopapular, but macules or papules may predominate. The lesions come and go on various sites on the trunk and limbs before they disappear permanently. The rash may become confluent and intensified in areas subject to irritation.

1.25

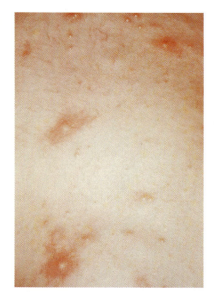

Figure 1.25. Close-up of the lesions in erythema toxicum neonatorum. The etiology is unknown but biopsy of the lesions show the presence of numerous eosinophils. It has been suggested that the presence of erythema toxicum is evidence of maturity.

1.26

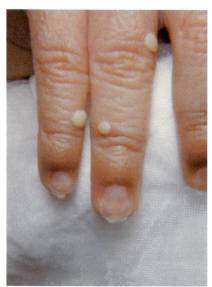 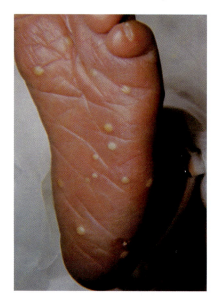

Figure 1.26. Erythema toxicum neonatorum may present as vesicular lesions, which were present at birth in this infant. Note the lack of inflammation surrounding the vesicles (which actually look like pustules). These lesions may be associated with the more usual maculopapular lesions elsewhere on the skin. The diagnosis of erythema toxicum was confirmed by examination of a stained smear from the lesions in which eosinophils alone were present and numerous. The vesicles resolved spontaneously. Differential diagnosis includes herpetic lesions and transient neonatal pustular melanosis.

1.27

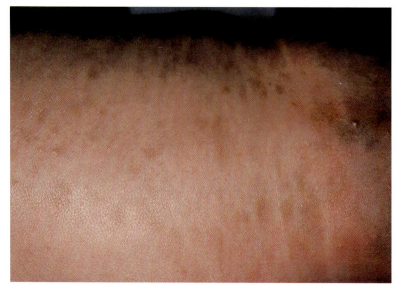

Figure 1.27. Lentigines are smooth, freckle-like, pigmented macules. They are usually present at birth, have a scattered distribution, and have been considered by some to be a manifestation of intrauterine erythema toxicum neonatorum. They usually disappear within 6 to 8 weeks.

1.28

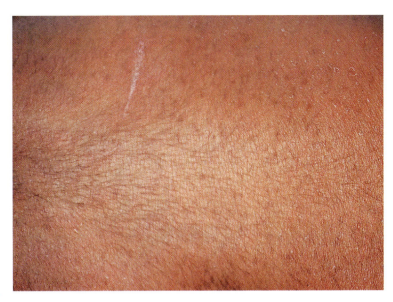

Figure 1.28. Another example of lentigines. Note the scattered distribution of the lesions which were present at birth. Lentigines should be differentiated from freckles (ephelides) which are red or light brown, well-circumscribed macules usually less than 5 mm in diameter. Freckles are not seen in infancy but appear in childhood, especially on sun-exposed areas of the skin. In general, freckles are found in clusters. Because they normally do not appear in the axilla, their presence in this area is a strong indication of neurofibromatosis.

1.29

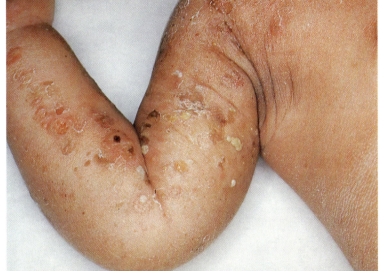

Figure 1.29. Transient neonatal pustular melanosis in an infant at the age of 3 days. This is a benign self-limiting disorder of unknown etiology characterized by superficial sterile vesiculopustular lesions that rupture early. They present as intact pustules as well as ruptured lesions which become evanescent hyperpigmented macules. These lesions are usually present at birth and are seen in 0.5 to 2% of newborns. Over 90% of the infants with this condition are black. The lesions are most often seen in clusters under the chin, and on the forehead, neck, lower back, and the extremities. They generally regress within 1 to 2 months and the hyperpigmented area eventually blends as the surrounding skin darkens.

1.30

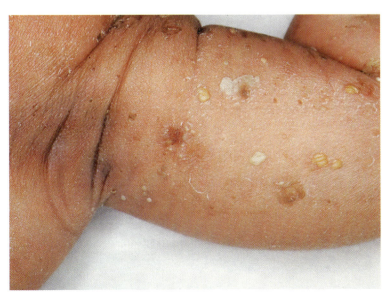

Figure 1.30. Another example of transient neonatal pustular melanosis in which the typical lesions are present. Note the vesiculopustular lesions and the brown hyperpigmented macules. The lesions of transient neonatal pustular melanosis are sterile on culture, and smears of fluid from the vesicles demonstrate neutrophils and cellular debris. There are few or no eosinophils, in contrast to the lesions of erythema toxicum neonatorum which reveal clusters of eosinophils and a relative absence of neutrophils. Differential diagnosis includes erythema toxicum and staphylococcal, herpetic, or candidal infections.

1.31

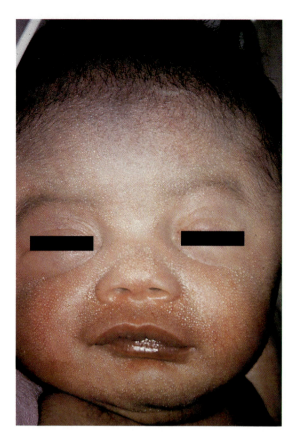

1.32

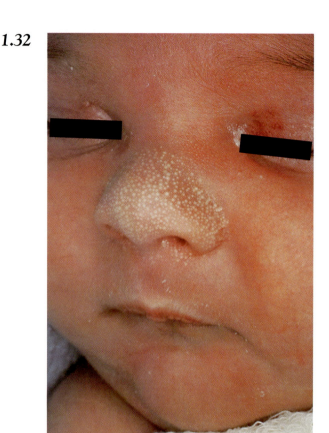

Figure 1.31. Sebaceous gland hyperplasia represents a physiologic phenomenon of the newborn manifested by multiple, yellow to flesh-colored tiny greasy-looking papules that occur on the nose, cheeks, and upper lips of full term infants. These papules, a manifestation of maternal androgen stimulation, represent a temporary disorder that resolves spontaneously within the first few weeks of life.

Figure 1.32. A close-up view of sebaceous gland hyperplasia.

1.33

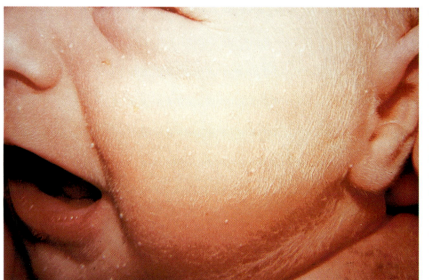

Figure 1.33. Milia occur commonly on the face of 25 to 40% of newborn infants. Histologically they are small superficial inclusion cysts that result from retention of keratin and sebaceous material within the pilosebaceous glands of the newborn, and appear as tiny 1- to 2-mm white or yellowish-white papules. The lesions are called "milia" because of their resemblance to millet seeds. Milia are particularly prominent on the cheeks, nose, chin, and nasolabial folds. The condition is self-limiting and resolves within the first month of life. Persistent and numerous milia may be seen in association with other defects (e.g., oral-facial-digital syndrome type I).

Figure 1.34. Miliaria crystallina (sudamina) consists of clear superficial pinpoint vesicles without an inflammatory areola. The lesions appear especially on the head and chest. Each vesicle is related to a sweat gland, the duct of which has been obstructed or occluded. The rash differs from milia in that the vesicles lack the white opacity of milia, generally appear a little later (in the 2nd week), and are often related to excessive warmth and humidity. The incidence is greatest in the first few weeks of life owing to the relative immaturity of the eccrine ducts which favor poral closure and sweat retention.

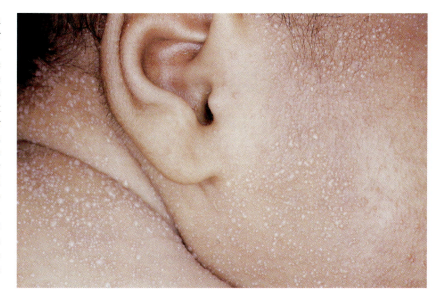

1.34

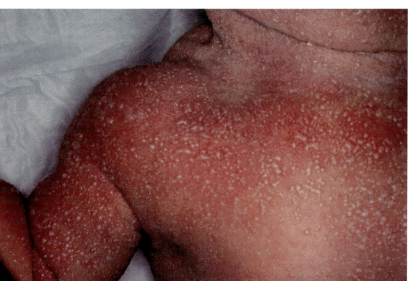

1.35

Figure 1.35. Miliaria rubra (prickly heat) is characterized by small discrete erythematous papules, vesicles, or papulovesicles which are surrounded by erythema. Lesions have a predilection for covered parts of the body where the baby gets overheated. It is important to unwrap these babies and avoid excessive heat.

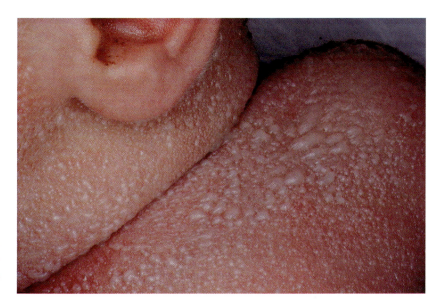

1.36

Figure 1.36. A close-up of the lesions of miliaria rubra. Note the clear vesicles and erythema of the surrounding skin.

1.37

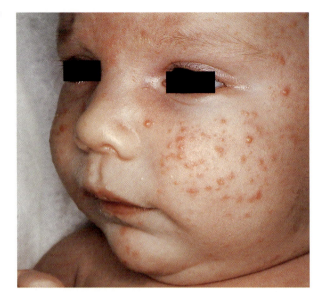

Figure 1.37. Infants with acne neonatorum have the typical facial distribution of the comedones seen in acne in adolescence. The chest and back are rarely involved. Neonatal acne appears to develop as a result of maternal androgen stimulation of sebaceous glands that have not yet involuted to their childhood state of immaturity. Acne neonatorum is a common, transitory, self-limiting disorder and should not be mistaken for an infection.

1.38

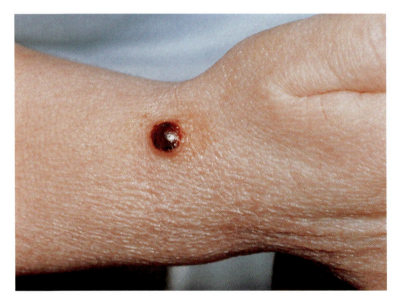

Figure 1.38. Intrauterine sucking lesions (sucking blisters) may present as small intact or ruptured bullae and are most commonly seen on the radial surface of the wrist, dorsum of the hand, or dorsum of the fingers. If unruptured, as in this infant, they may be filled with sterile serous fluid or, if sucking is vigorous, there may be a hemorrhagic component. Intrauterine sucking lesions are an example of self-induced tissue disruption in a normal newborn; the lesions are benign and require no therapy.

1.39

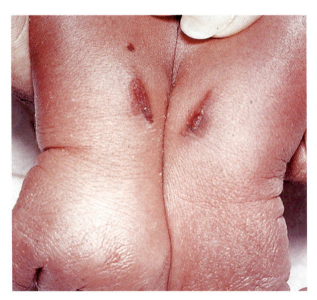

Figure 1.39. The intrauterine sucking lesions at the wrists in this infant have ruptured and left raw areas which will not heal as long as the infant continues sucking at the site.

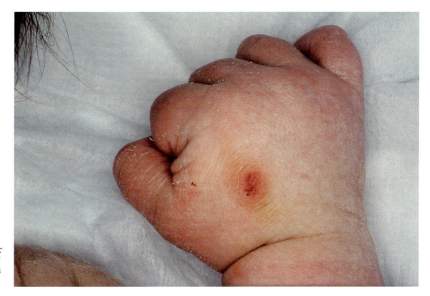

1.40

Figure 1.40. Another example of an intrauterine sucking lesion on the dorsum of the right hand.

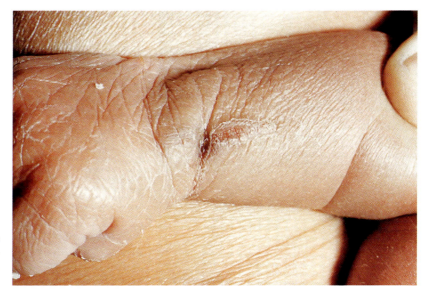

1.41

Figure 1.41. The intrauterine sucking lesions may heal and present at birth with an area of scarring, as noted in this infant.

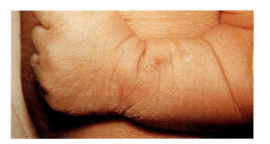

1.42

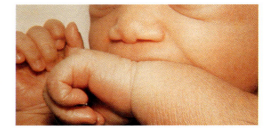

Figure 1.42. In upper panel, note another example of scarring at the left wrist in a normal newborn from an intrauterine sucking lesion. Below, this infant continued sucking its wrist after birth at the site of this lesion.

1.43

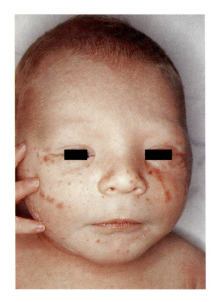

Figure 1.43. Facial abrasions in this infant were self-inflicted. This type of lesion results from hyperactivity in an infant with long finger nails and is seen more commonly in postmature infants and in infants with drug withdrawal.

1.44

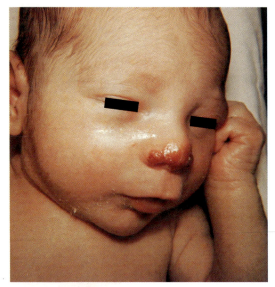

Figure 1.44. Abrasion of the nose ("sheet burns") in an infant with hyperactivity due to drug withdrawal. At the present time hyperactivity is most commonly seen with drug withdrawal, but may occur in infants experiencing pain, congenital hyperthyroidism, etc. The abrasions and erythema generally develop over prominent body parts such as the nose, ears, cheeks, elbows, and knees.

1.45

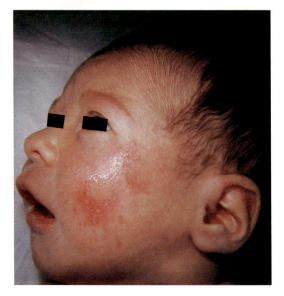

Figure 1.45. "Sheet burn" of the cheeks in a hyperactive infant who was lying in a pool of regurgitated gastric contents. A similar appearance could occur with hyperactivity in an infant with drug **withdrawal alone.**

1.46

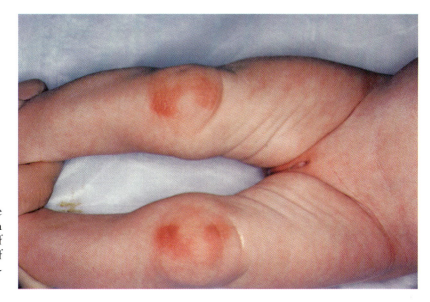

Figure 1.46. Abrasions of the knees occurring in an infant with drug withdrawal. This type of lesion, which occurs as a result of repeated hip flexion in a hyperactive infant, is very common.

1.47

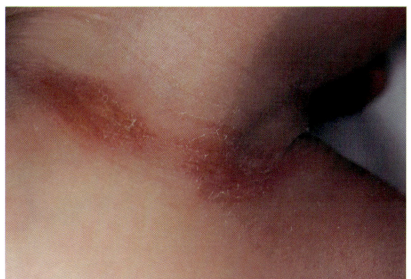

Figure 1.47. This infant presented at birth with an abraded area in the neck. The cord was around the neck three times and this was thought to be the etiology of the abrasion.

1.48

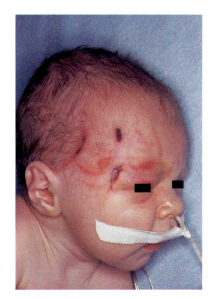

Figure 1.48. The abrasions of the head and face in this normal infant occurred with forceps delivery. There was rapid healing.

1.49

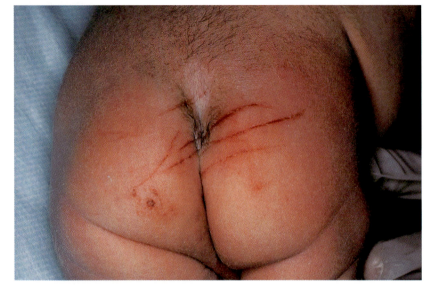

Figure 1.49. Skin incisions over the buttocks in an infant following cesarean birth.

1.50

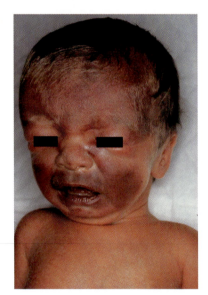

Figure 1.50. Edema and ecchymoses of the face in a premature infant who was delivered as a face presentation. These infants need to be checked for anemia and hyperbilirubinemia.

1.51

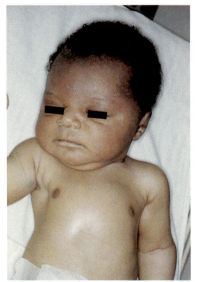

Figure 1.51. Suffusion of the face and head in an infant who had a tight nuchal cord. Note the difference in color of the face and head compared with the rest of the body.

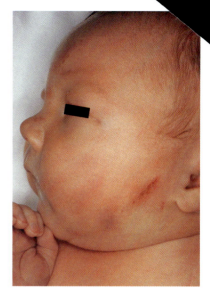

Figure 1.52. In this infant aged 6 days, note the healing abrasion from the application of forceps. In addition note the changes in the skin in that there is some reddish-purple discoloration and swelling with induration of the underlying subcutaneous tissue. This is an example of early subcutaneous fat necrosis. Subcutaneous fat necrosis occurs in areas subjected to undue pressure such as by forceps.

1.53

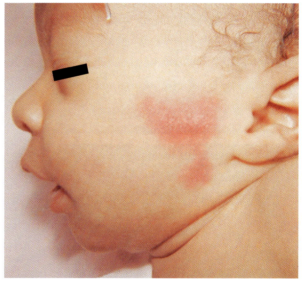

Figure 1.53. Subcutaneous fat necrosis of the cheek in an infant following forceps delivery. In subcutaneous fat necrosis, which is usually detected towards the end of the first week of life, the lesions have an inflammatory or ecchymotic appearance. The underlying tissue may be indurated and feels diffusely hardened. With breakdown of the subcutaneous tissue after several days there may be an area in the center which is fluctuant. If managed conservatively, spontaneous healing usually occurs. This condition should not be mistakenly treated as an infection.

1.54

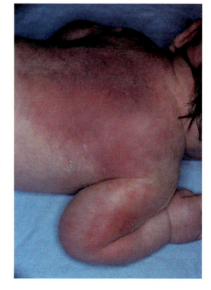

Figure 1.54. This infant, aged 5 days and delivered as a breech presentation, developed the extensive reddish-purple discoloration and swelling of the skin over the back with induration of the underlying subcutaneous tissue. This is an example of extensive subcutaneous fat necrosis. With conservative treatment, improvement occurred within 2 to 3 weeks.

Differential diagnosis includes sclerema neonatorum in which there is progressive hardening of the subcutaneous tissue associated with severe illness of the infant. In sclerema the involved areas are hard and non-pitting and the palms and soles are spared.

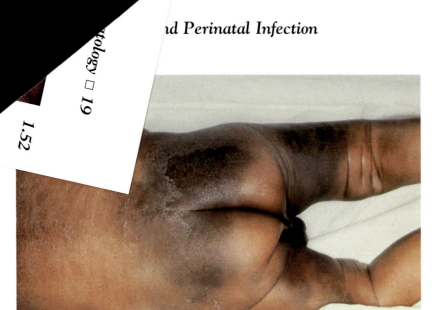

Figure 1.55. During delivery of this infant with a breech presentation there was much manipulation and handling. He developed severe generalized subcutaneous fat necrosis which presented as numerous ecchymotic lesions with marked induration of the skin. Any handling of this infant resulted in pain and discomfort. Over a period of several weeks the subcutaneous fat necrosis improved but the infant developed hypercalcemia. His serum calcium level was 15.8 mg/dL. (There is a case report of an infant with subcutaneous fat necrosis who developed a serum calcium level of greater than 20 mg/dL.)

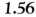

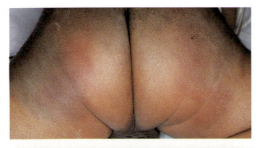

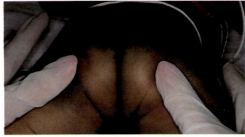

Figure 1.56. This infant delivered by emergency cesarean birth was an extremely difficult delivery and on the 4th day of life he developed an area of subcutaneous fat necrosis over each buttock as noted in the top panel. In the lower panel, note how pressure over these sites during delivery resulted in the subcutaneous fat necrosis.

1.57

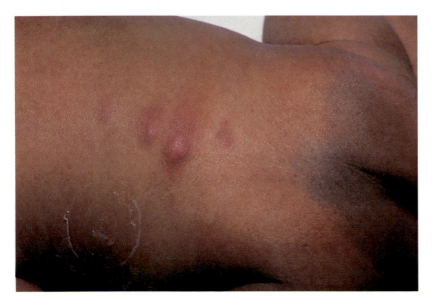

Figure 1.57. In this infant there were several attempts at performing a spinal tap for sepsis evaluation. Four days later he developed areas of subcutaneous fat necrosis over the lower lumbar area. These could easily have been mistaken for abscesses but were confirmed to be subcutaneous fat necrosis occurring from the pressure applied in performing the spinal tap. Note the mongolian spots.

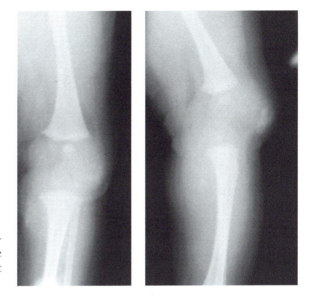

1.58

Figure 1.58. Calcification may occur in areas of subcutaneous fat necrosis. In this radiograph note the soft tissue calcifications occurring as a result of subcutaneous fat necrosis.

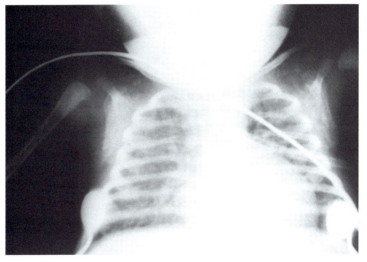

1.59

Figure 1.59. Calcifications occurred in the scapular area of this small premature infant as a result of subcutaneous fat necrosis which developed from vigorous chest physiotherapy.

DEVELOPMENTAL ABNORMALITIES OF THE SKIN

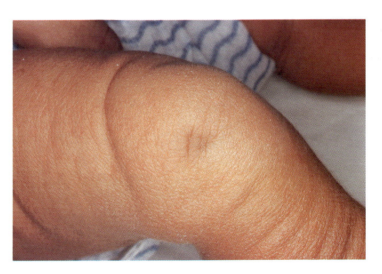

1.60

Figure 1.60. This infant has a typical pigmented skin dimple at the knee. The presence of a skin dimple over a joint, pigmented or not, is normal. Skin dimpling is frequently noted in a relatively mild form where there has been prolonged intrauterine pressure upon the bony prominences, particularly at the elbows and knees. Normal skin dimples are most commonly noted at the knee joints, over the lateral aspect of the elbows, over the acromion process, and in the lumbosacral area.

1.61

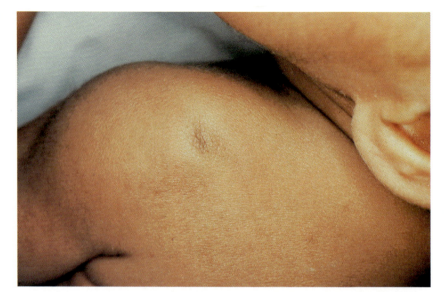

Figure 1.61. A pigmented skin dimple over the left shoulder. Normal skin dimples in general tend to occur in areas where the skin is relatively tightly bound to the underlying bony prominences.

1.62

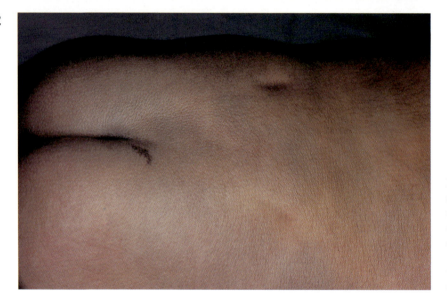

Figure 1.62. Nonpigmented skin dimples in the iliosacral area. These tend to be crease-shaped and may be multiple over the lower part of the back. If midline, they should be distinguished from a pilonidal sinus.

1.63

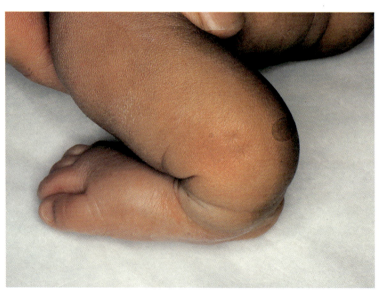

Figure 1.63. Dimples in between the joints over the long bones are considered pathologic until proven otherwise. In this infant with congenital hypophosphatasia, the skin dimple over the middle of the tibia is a very typical finding. Abnormal (aberrant) skin dimples may occur at a location where there has been a closer than usual proximity between the skin and the underlying bone structure during fetal life, resulting in deficient development of subcutaneous tissue at that locus. Such dimples may be secondary either to a loss of subcutaneous tissue or to an aberrant bony promontory. These may also cause breakdown of the dermis with ulcer formation.

1.64

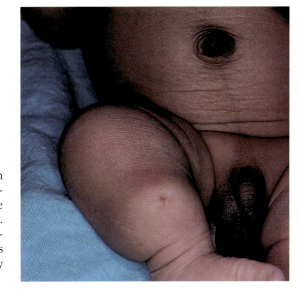

Figure 1.64. An example of an abnormal skin dimple in an infant with camptomelic dysplasia. Note the extreme prenatal distortion of the bones with the development of the aberrant skin dimples over the abnormal bony prominences. The most common site for this type of abnormal skin dimple is over the apex of a severe curvature of the tibia in cases of fibular hypoplasia, but other areas can be similarly affected.

1.65

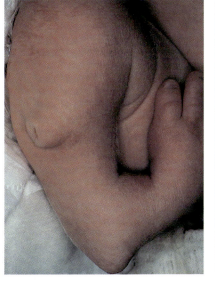

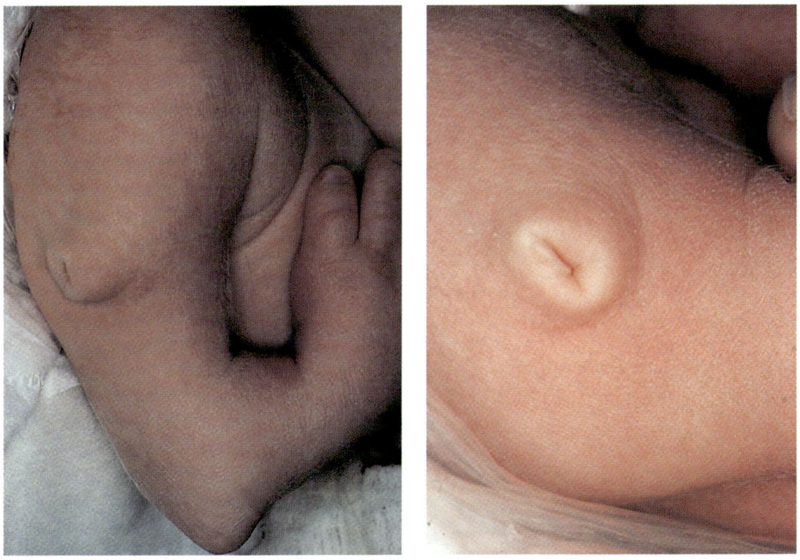

Figure 1.65. This infant with exstrophy of the cloaca sequence had a dysplastic, markedly hypoplastic right tibia with deformity of the right foot. Note the severity of the abnormal skin dimple.

1.66

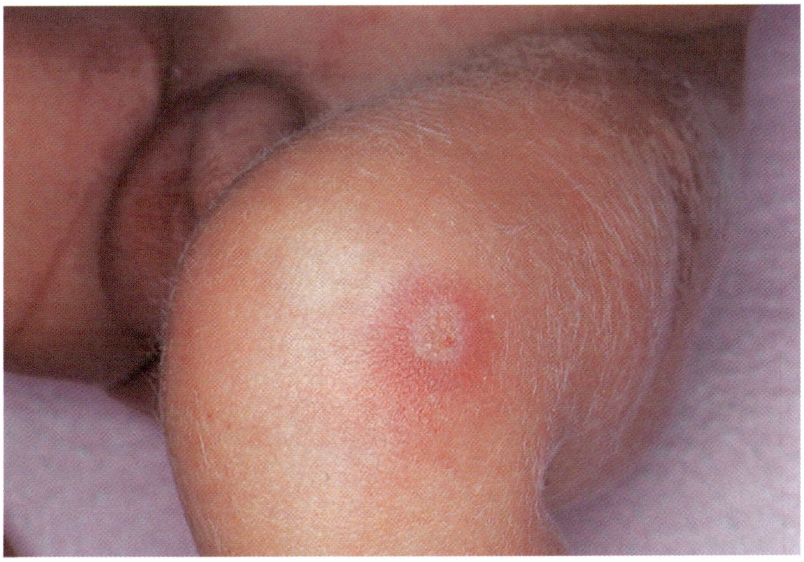

Figure 1.66. Ulceration of the skin, which was present at birth in this infant, occurred as a result of intrauterine pressure on the fetus.

1.67

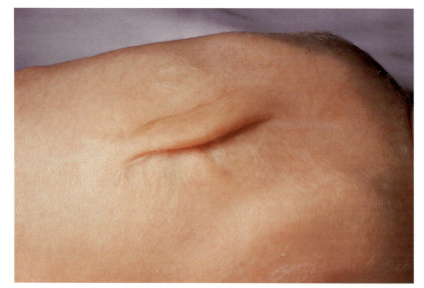

Figure 1.67. The large skin fold on the back of this infant was hard and fibrotic. It was believed to have occurred as a result of the skin being "pinched" in utero from intrauterine constraint very early in gestation.

1.68

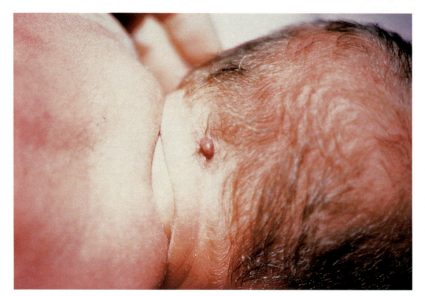

Figure 1.68. A midline occipital defect consisting of a tag with some cystic formation is seen in this infant. In any infant with a midline lesion anywhere from the back of the neck to the lower end of the spine, it is mandatory to investigate the neural axis. The lesions may consist of small sinuses, cysts, or hemangiomas.

1.69

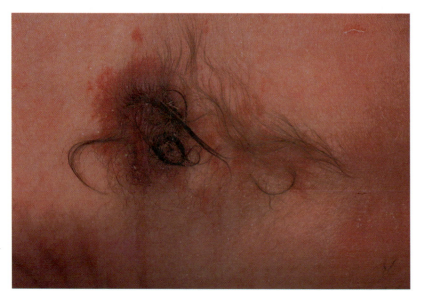

Figure 1.69. This infant presented with a midline hemangioma associated with a midline tuft of hair over the spine. Further investigation confirmed the presence of a neural axis defect. If hair tufts are associated with any of these lesions, the risk is even greater.

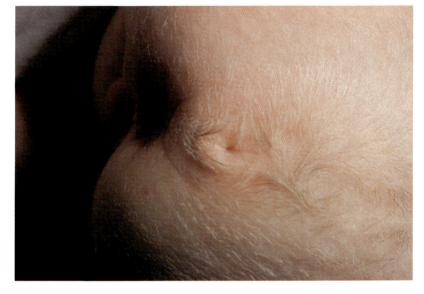

1.70

Figure 1.70. Pilonidal dimples are extremely common in neonates. If the base of the dimple can be seen easily, further investigation is not necessary. If the dimple is very deep or appears to be a sinus tract it is important to do a neurologic evaluation.

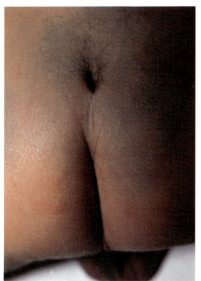

1.71

Figure 1.71. Another example of a pilonidal dimple which is deep. This infant's MRI study was normal.

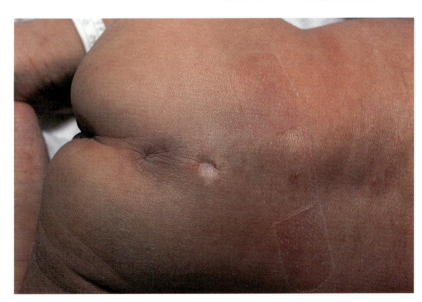

1.72

Figure 1.72. In this infant there is a midline defect over the distal end of the spine. With this type of lesion it is mandatory to do further studies. MRI confirmed the presence of a tethered cord syndrome. Note the "bandaid sign" in this infant confirming that the infant had a spinal tap performed as part of a sepsis evaluation. This was contraindicated in this infant because of the midline skin defect.

1.73

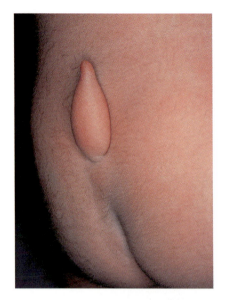 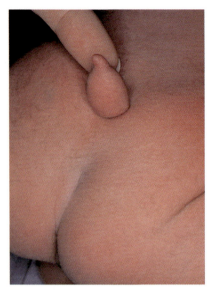

Figure 1.73. A baby with a tail. Vestigial tails are rarely seen in the neonate. They may consist of soft tissue only, as in this infant, or may contain osseous structures.

1.74

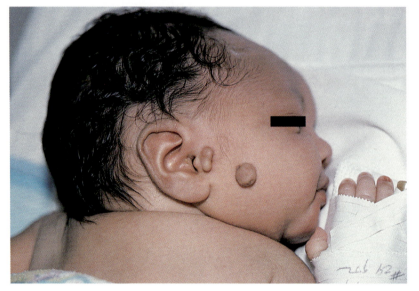

Figure 1.74. Note the preauricular and facial skin tags in this otherwise normal infant. Preauricular skin tags are extremely common, but the presence of skin tags between the ear and corner of the mouth would suggest a diagnosis of Goldenhar's syndrome.

1.75

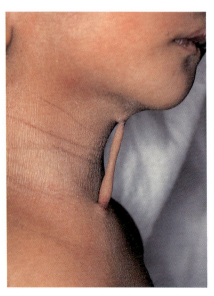 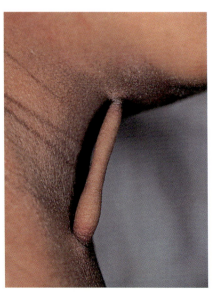

Figure 1.75. Midline skin and tissue band between the jaw and lower sternum in an otherwise normal infant.

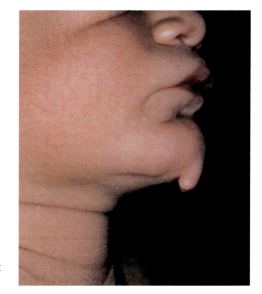

1.76

Figure 1.76. A midline skin tag of the chin. This consisted of soft tissue only. The radiograph of the mandible was normal.

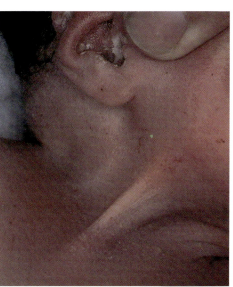

1.77

Figure 1.77. This infant has redundancy of the skin in the neck which was present at birth. It was related to the infant's position in utero in that the head was flexed on the right upper chest, resulting in the tight skin. There may be a small amount of redundant skin in the neck normally, but when there is enough to cause visible folds or webs on the lateral neck, prenatal edema in the region is almost certain to be the cause. Extensive redundancy of neck skin is seen in a number of dysmorphic conditions (e.g., Turner's and Noonan's syndromes). Once localized skin growth has taken place, it does not easily reconstitute itself if the distending forces are removed.

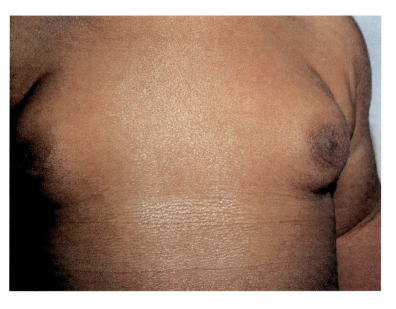

1.78

Figure 1.78. Mastitis neonatorum due to physiologic breast engorgement is the result of transplacental transfer of maternal estrogen to the fetus. Enlargement is generally symmetrical, as noted in this infant. Witch's milk (which is chemically identical to colostrum) may be expressed from the breasts, but it is not advisable to relieve the swelling by expressing the milk since infection may follow.

1.79

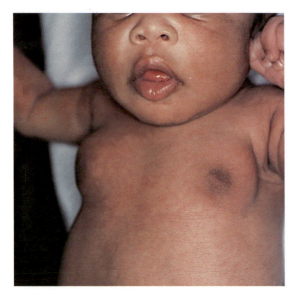

Figure 1.79. Another example of mastitis neonatorum which is asymmetrical in that it is more prominent on the right than on the left. Mastitis neonatorum is noted more frequently in postmature infants. It subsides spontaneously over the course of several weeks.

1.80

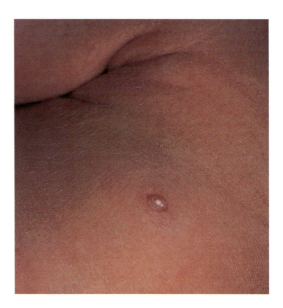

Figure 1.80. This infant has inclusion cysts of the right nipple. These require no treatment as they resolve spontaneously.

1.81

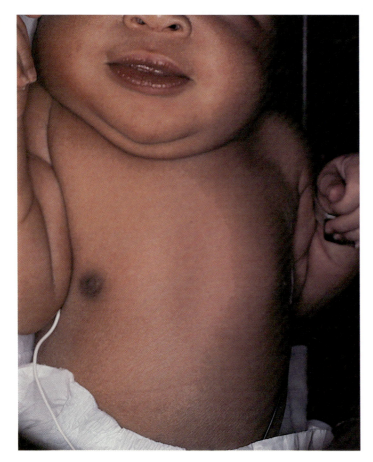

Figure 1.81. Note that the nipples are in the 5th intercostal space in this otherwise normal infant. The nipple may be found anywhere along the milk line which extends from the axilla to the pubis. Normally the nipple is located at the 4th intercostal space.

1.82

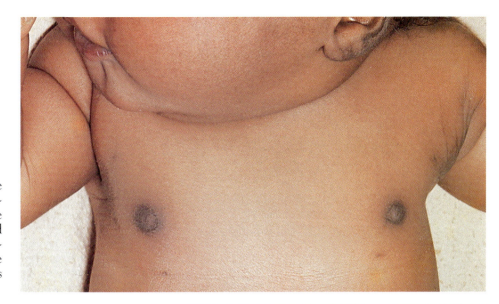

Figure 1.82. Note the bilateral supernumerary nipples in the anterior axilla and bilateral supernumerary nipples below the normal nipples in this black infant.

1.83

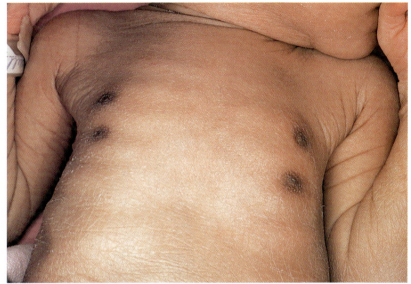

Figure 1.83. Supernumerary nipples are especially common in members of darkly pigmented racial groups. They occur anywhere along the milk line and the supernumerary breast tissue may present as an oval pigmented spot less than half the size of the normal nipple, or may present as another fully developed nipple.

1.84

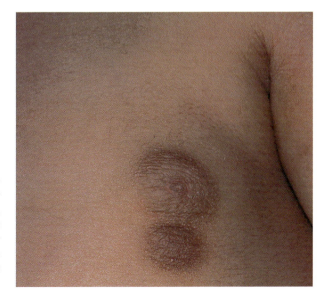

Figure 1.84. In this infant there is a unilateral supernumerary breast on the left side. Supernumerary breasts are rare. These are potentially functional and, like extra nipples, these structures occur along the embryonic milk line unilaterally or bilaterally, usually below the normal site of breast placement. The nipple and areola are quite well developed, distinguishing this anomaly from simple supernumerary nipples.

1.85

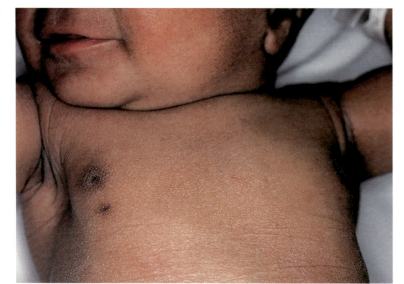

Figure 1.85. Note that the nipples are wide-spaced and there is a right-sided unilateral supernumerary nipple. In general, wide-spaced nipples occur rarely in infants with a normal chest configuration. Infants with Turner's or Noonan's syndrome have wide-spaced nipples but have a shield-like chest.

1.86

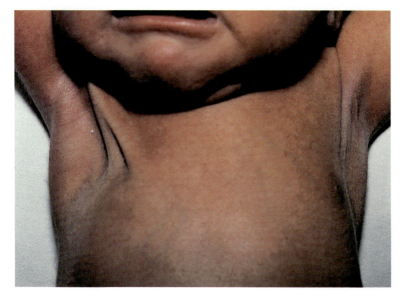

Figure 1.86. This infant with Poland's anomaly has absence of the nipple (athelia) on the right associated with the absence of the pectoralis muscle. Athelia is rare but is seen unilaterally in infants with Poland's anomaly, and bilaterally in certain forms of ectodermal dysplasia.

Hypoplastic nipples are usually poorly pigmented with a narrow or absent areolar zone and little palpable breast tissue. Both sides are equally affected. Absence of the breast (amastia) is very rare. There is no sign of nipple, areola, or mammary tissue.

1.87

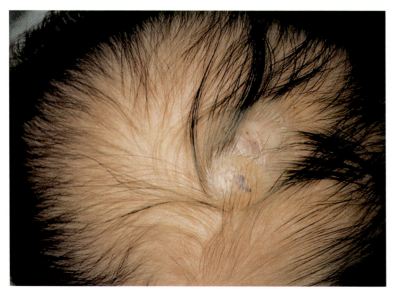

Figure 1.87. Congenital scalp defect (aplasia cutis congenita) occurs most commonly as a single small defect of the scalp, 1 to 2 cm across, and is usually located close to the normal site of a parietal hair whorl. The lesions have a well defined edge with a punched-out appearance, and may be multiple or involve a larger portion of the scalp. Etiology is unknown, and they heal with scarring leaving a zone of permanent alopecia.

1.88

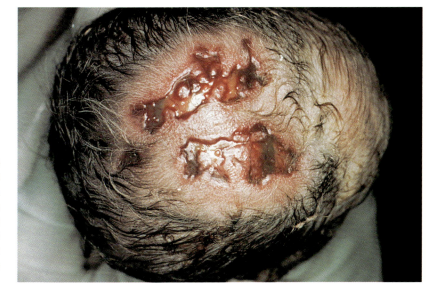

Figure 1.88. Scalp defects are a frequent finding in infants with trisomy 13, as in this infant. A more severe congenital scalp defect may have a full thickness absence of the skin with large areas of skin aplasia. This lesion may occur as a result of in utero disruption by an amniotic band.

1.89

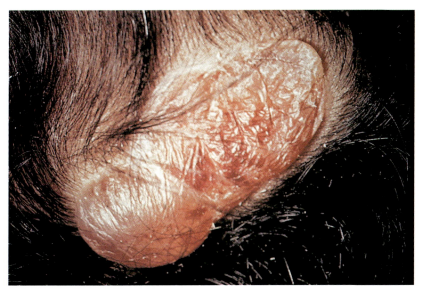

Figure 1.89. In this otherwise normal infant there is a large congenital scalp defect associated with a bullous bleb.

1.90

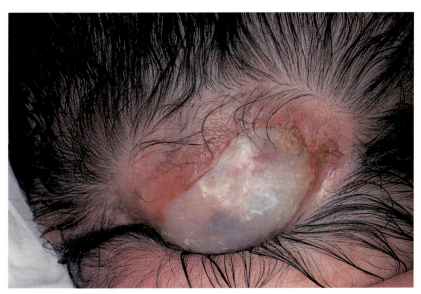

Figure 1.90. A massive congenital scalp defect which involved the skull and exposed the dura mater.

1.91

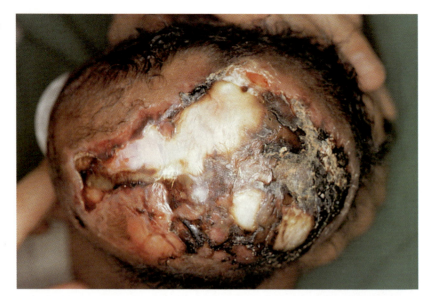

Figure 1.91. The severe congenital scalp defect in this infant occurred in the Adams-Oliver syndrome, which is a disruption sequence associated with limb reduction anomalies and scalp and skin defects as a result of amniotic bands.

1.92

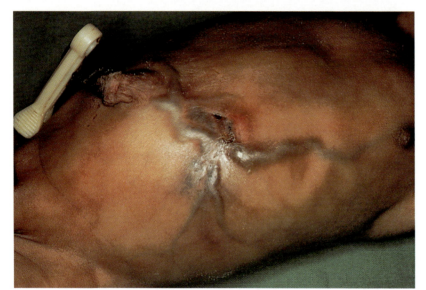

Figure 1.92. The same infant showing the marked aplasia cutis congenita in the skin of the abdomen with dilated superficial capillaries. This is an example of aplasia of the skin affecting the trunk as a result of amniotic bands. It is quite rare.

1.93

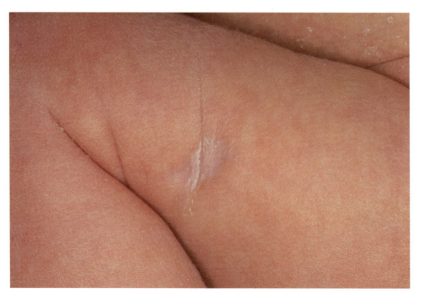

Figure 1.93. Congenital skin defect of the thigh in an infant. It is not known whether this type of disruption results from an intrinsic abnormality of the skin itself or whether aberrant bands of amniotic tissue adhere to intact fetal skin. Some cases of scarring of the skin, especially if linear, have been associated with prenatal varicella infections.

1.94

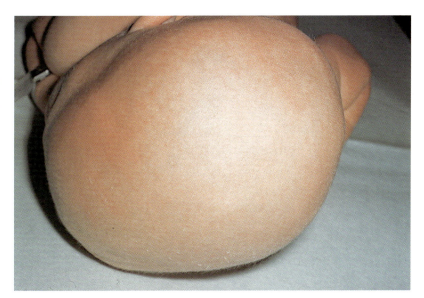

Figure 1.94. Congenital alopecia is usually an autosomal recessive disorder but may be an isolated event. Hair development begins at about week 14 of gestation, and from gestational week 20 until birth the body is covered with fine lanugo hair. This is gradually replaced during the first months of postnatal life with coarser, moderately pigmented vellus hair. Alopecia or hypotrichosis occurs in several syndromes (e.g., ectodermal dysplasia where the hair is sparse over the scalp, eyebrows, and eyelashes; progeria; Hallermann-Streiff syndrome; and cartilage-hair hypoplasia).

1.95

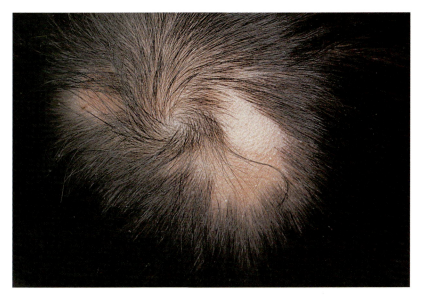

Figure 1.95. The scalp of this infant showed a patchy alopecia at birth. A hair whorl is situated over the part of the brain growing most rapidly from about 16 to 19 weeks of gestation. The normal position is slightly lateral to the midline in the posterior parietal zone. It appears that this patch of alopecia is related to this. Physiologic "frictional" alopecia usually occurs over the occipital region as a result of head rolling and friction producing hair loss on the back of the head. It is poorly circumscribed and resolves completely once the infant is able to change its position at will.

1.96

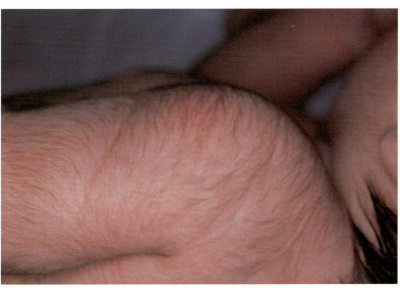

Figure 1.96. Hypertrichosis is seen in normal infants, especially in hispanic infants who tend to have more hair than caucasian or black infants. In hispanics especially there may be hairy ears with long coarse dark hair emerging from the lateral and posterior surface of the pinna.

1.97

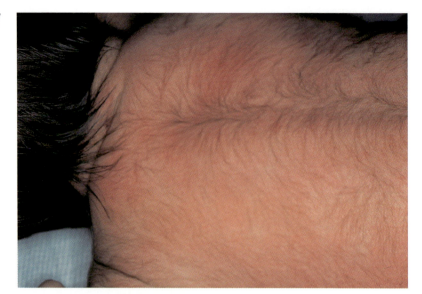

Figure 1.97. Hypertrichosis in a Hispanic infant whose mother was an epileptic treated with phenytoin throughout her pregnancy. Hypertrichosis is associated with syndromes such as Cornelia de Lange's, leprechaunism, etc. In infants with hypertrichosis associated with syndromes, there may be a low anterior hairline which is especially noted at the sides of the forehead approaching the lateral eyebrows due to a widened "sideburn."

1.98

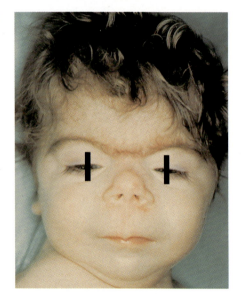

Figure 1.98. Hypertrichosis in an infant with Cornelia de Lange's syndrome. Note also the synophrys, anteverted nostrils, and lack of philtrum. Synophrys (bridging of the eyebrows in the midline) is seen in Cornelia de Lange's syndrome, Waardenburg's syndrome, and in otherwise normal infants. The skin between the eyebrows usually bears only fine vellus hairs, and when the brows encroach on this area they produce the appearance of a single band of hair above the eyes. Straight eyelashes emerge from the lid margin at a steep angle and extend straight downward rather than exhibiting the gentle upward curve. Such eyelashes are seen in children with severe neuromuscular disease and may be caused by lack of normal muscle tone in the levator palpebri superioris muscle.

1.99

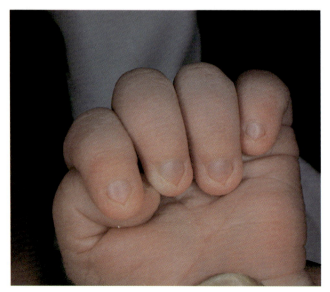

Figure 1.99. This infant's triangular nails fit into the category of tapered nails that become progressively narrower and more hyperconvex as they grow distally. The nails generally reflect the size and shape of the underlying distal phalanx (e.g., hypoplastic nail, narrow hyperconvex nail, short broad nail).

1.100

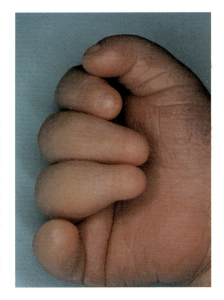
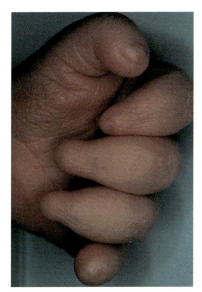

Figure 1.100. In this infant with the fetal hydantoin syndrome the nails are hypoplastic and distorted or absent over the short hypoplastic distal phalanges. Note the digitalization of the thumbs. Total nail aplasia is very rare. At birth, some or all of the fingers bear a rudimentary nail bed. In nail-patella syndrome, partial nail aplasia occurs, particularly in the thumbs and index fingers.

1.101

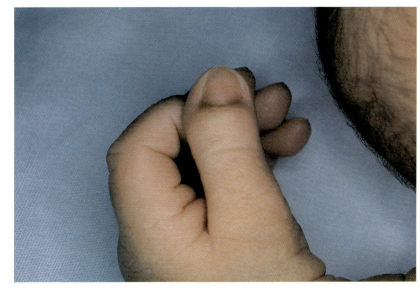

Figure 1.101. Unusually broad nails of normal length are found over digits with duplication of the distal phalanx. They are also seen in Rubenstein-Taybi syndrome and Larsen's syndrome.

1.102

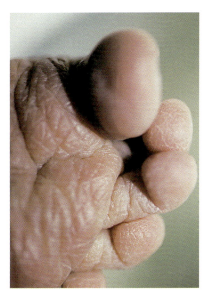
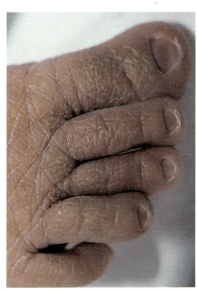

Figure 1.102. Unusually broad toes in another infant with Rubenstein-Taybi syndrome.

VASCULAR DISORDERS AND MALFORMATIONS

1.103

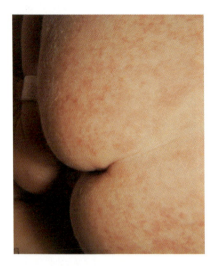

Figure 1.103. Petechiae are common in normal infants, particularly over the back and buttocks. They usually disappear within a few days. Facial petechiae are commonly seen in infants in whom there was a nuchal cord or where there was abnormal delay following delivery of the head and neck before the trunk and shoulders were delivered.

1.104

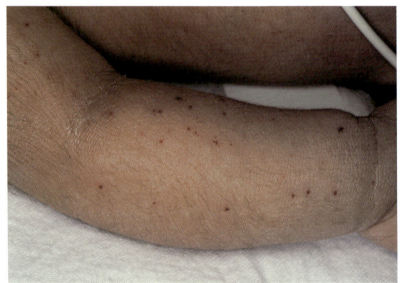

Figure 1.104. The petechiae in this infant were associated with severe birth asphyxia. The platelet count was 90,000/mm³ and the petechiae resolved spontaneously within a few days.

1.105

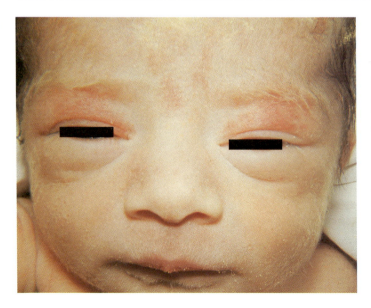

Figure 1.105. Macular hemangioma ("angel's kiss") of the eyelids in a newborn infant. Vascular nevi occur in up to 40% of newborns. They are divided into three groups (salmon patches, hemangiomas, and vascular malformations) and are classified by their histology and the degree of involvement of the skin and subcutaneous tissues. The most common are the salmon patches (macular hemangioma, nevus flammeus). They consist of dilated capillaries in the superficial layers of the dermis and are noted most commonly on the face, the midforehead, the glabella, philtrum, and the nape of the neck. Multiple sites are often affected.

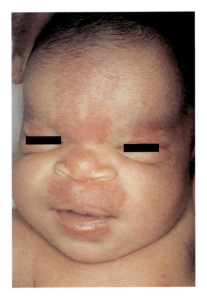

Figure 1.106. Macular hemangioma of the eyelids, glabella, and face. Macular hemangiomas (telangiectatic nevi) are poorly defined, bright red in color, and blanch easily with pressure, but the blood returns rapidly. In general these capillary hemangiomas become less visible in the first year of life as the skin becomes less translucent.

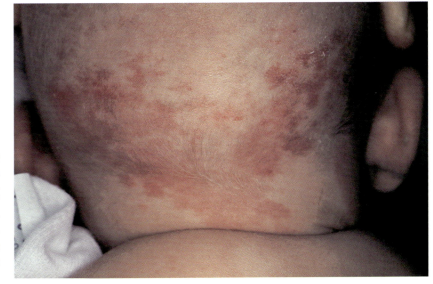

Figure 1.107. A macular hemangioma (salmon patch) in the nape of the neck is commonly called the "stork-bite" nevus. These are the most common of the macular hemangiomas and fade gradually, but are more likely to persist than other macular hemangiomas.

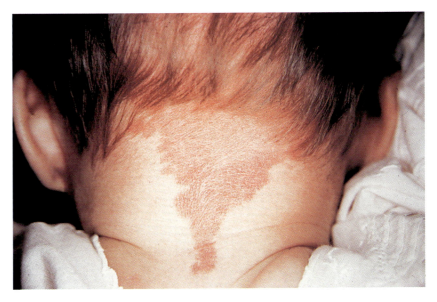

Figure 1.108. An infant at age 5 months with a "stork-bite" nevus.

1.109

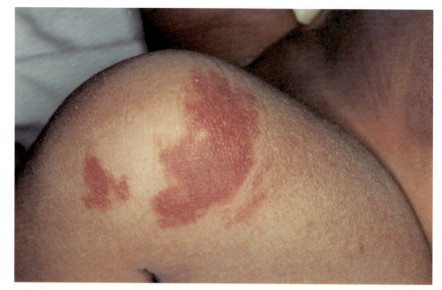

Figure 1.109. A macular hemangioma of the left knee in an infant. Lesions on the trunk and limbs may be extensive.

1.110

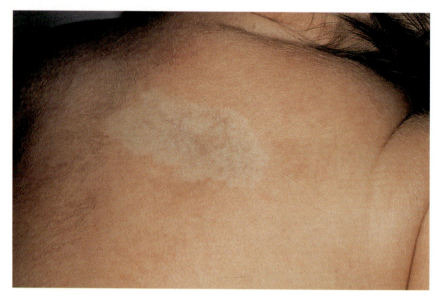

Figure 1.110. A nevus anemicus present at birth on the back of an infant. Note that the nevus is pale and has prominent capillaries. It may be the precursor of a strawberry nevus in that it starts as a fine, thread-like telangiectasis surrounded by an area of localized pallor. Both strawberry nevus and nevus anemicus involute spontaneously.

1.111

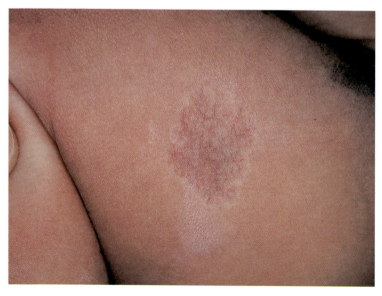

Figure 1.111. Another example of a nevus anemicus present at birth on the left thigh. Capillary hemangiomas (strawberry nevi) may be present at birth, but generally develop during the first few postnatal weeks as pale or slightly reddened, well-demarcated zones of skin a few millimeters to several centimeters in diameter. They may occur on any area of the body but are seen most commonly on the head and neck (40%) and the trunk (30%). During the first months of life, rapid growth occurs and the lesions become elevated above the surrounding skin with a spongy consistency, and attain a bright red to purple color. Although compressible, they blanch with gentle pressure but seldom empty completely.

1.112

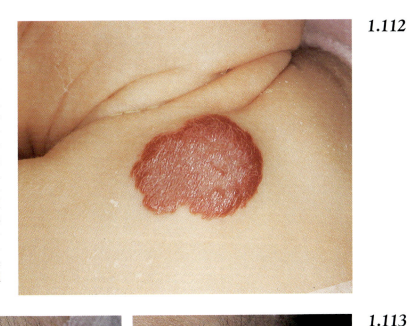

Figure 1.112. A capillary hemangioma (strawberry nevus) which developed in the upper thoracic region over the course of several weeks after birth is noted in this infant at the age of 3 weeks. The irregular surface with sharp demarcation is typical of a "strawberry" hemangioma which consists of dilated new capillaries in the dermal or subdermal area. The classic strawberry hemangioma is a raised, bright- or purplish-red lobulated tumor with well-defined borders and minute capillaries protruding from its surface, hence its "strawberry-like" appearance. Their history is usually one of continued rapid enlargement during the first few months of life followed by gradual spontaneous regression which occurs by central involution without scarring. In 50% of cases they resolve by the age of 5 years, in 70% by the age of 7 years, and in 90% by the age of 9 years.

1.113

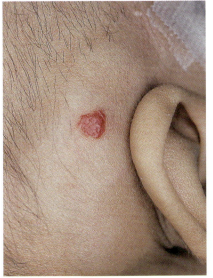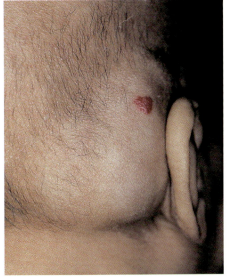

Figure 1.113. In this two and a half months old infant with a birthweight of 585 g, note the small strawberry nevus (figure left). This vascular tumor is apparently caused by a local persistence of angioblastic cells that give rise to a plexus of thin-walled capillaries with poor venous drainage. This continued to enlarge and at the age of three and one half months, note the marked enlargement of the nevus in the underlying tissue (figure right).

1.114

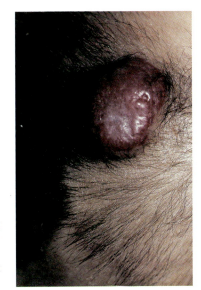

Figure 1.114. This 8-week-old premature infant with a birthweight of 900 g developed several strawberry nevi on the scalp at the age of 6 weeks. Note the rapid growth over a 2 week period. Hemangiomas are rarely seen in premature babies with a gestational age of less than 34 weeks. As the infant becomes older, hemangiomas may develop.

1.115

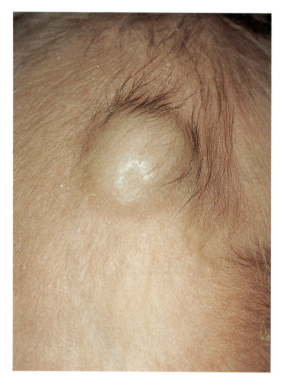

1.116

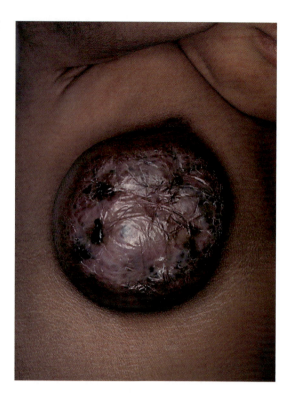

Figure 1.115. This infant shown in Figure 1.114, now at the age of 3 months, developed a cystic swelling over the scalp in the first few weeks of life. The cystic swelling increased gradually in size; note the bluish hue. On removal this was confirmed to be a strawberry hemangioma. Note that strawberry hemangiomas may have a large component visible on the surface of the skin, or may be covered by the skin, thus obscuring their characteristic appearance.

Figure 1.116. In some infants the lesion may appear to be a hemangioma but, as in this example, on biopsy the diagnosis was a hemangioendothelioma of the right chest.

1.117

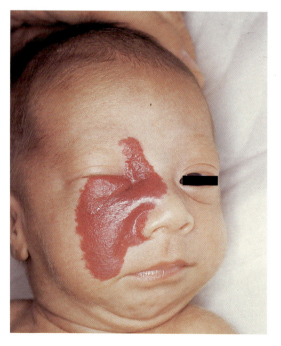

Figure 1.117. The capillary hemangioma involving the right side of the face in this infant demonstrates the fact that hemangiomas may expand sufficiently to interfere with function or may evidence bleeding or superficial infection. In this infant there would be marked interference with development of normal vision and, if untreated, this would lead to astigmatism and other problems. In such instances, treatment with steroids or laser surgery may be indicated.

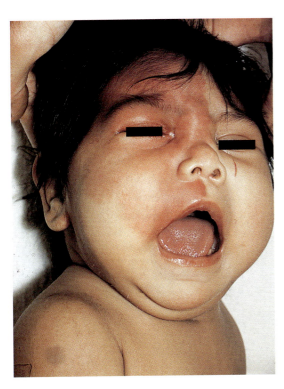

1.118

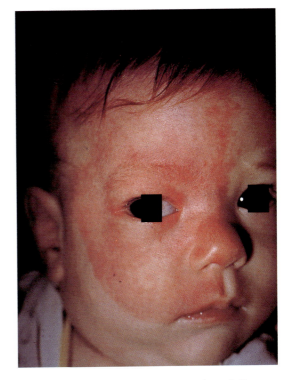

1.119

Figure 1.118. Port wine stain (nevus flammeus) is another macular hemangioma which represents a regional dilatation and enlargement of mature capillaries. It usually affects the skin of the face and neck, and the lesions are sharp-bordered and range in color from pale purple to deep burgundy. It usually does not indicate underlying abnormalities unless it extends into the area of distribution of the ophthalmic branch of the trigeminal nerve that serves the facial skin over the eyelid and up into the brow where, as in this infant, it may signal the presence of the intracranial vascular anomalies of Sturge-Weber syndrome (encephalotrigeminal angiomatosis).

Figure 1.119. Another example of Sturge-Weber syndrome in which the distribution involves both the 1st and 2nd branch of the trigeminal nerve. Note the glaucoma of the right eye. In Sturge-Weber syndrome, lesions stop at the midline. When extensive facial involvement is present, there may be an associated glaucoma (buphthalmos). As this is one of the neurocutaneous syndromes, a CT scan of the head should be done to exclude intracranial involvement. Radiographs of the skull may reveal unilateral curvilinear, double-contoured lines of calcification in the cerebral cortex ("railroad track calcification"). The intracerebral vascular abnormalities lead to brain atrophy and ocular lesions (optic atrophy).

Figure 1.120. This infant with involvement of the trunk and limbs is another example of Sturge-Weber syndrome. There were bilateral congenital glaucoma, seizures at the age of 6 days, and an abnormal CT scan. In Sturge-Weber syndrome, seizures occur in 80% of infants, mental retardation in a high percentage, and an associated glaucoma in 40 to 50% of the infants, especially if both the ophthalmic and maxillary branches of the trigeminal nerve are involved.

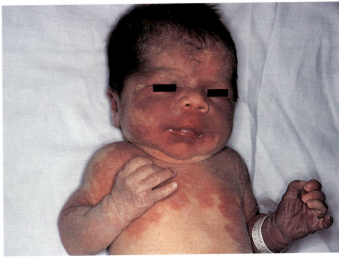

1.120

1.121

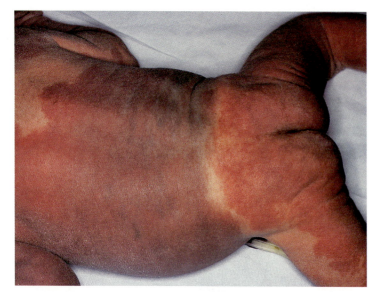

Figure 1.121. Note the widespread involvement of the trunk and limbs in the same infant. The likelihood of Sturge-Weber syndrome is greater when nevi such as these are present on the trunk and the limbs.

1.122

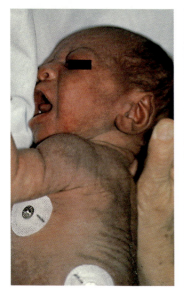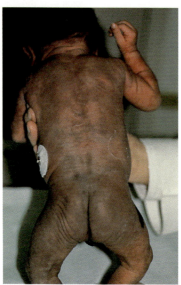

Figure 1.122. Phacomatosis pigmentovascularis is a rare condition in which there is a port wine appearance (as in Sturge-Weber syndrome) in addition to patches of slate-gray hyperpigmentation which clinically resemble mongolian spots. The infant also had a glaucoma of the left eye. This condition has been associated with glaucoma, seizures, and skeletal abnormalities.

1.123

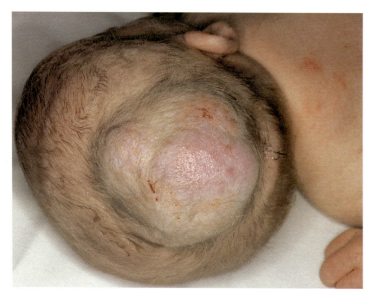

Figure 1.123. A large cavernous hemangioma was present on the scalp of this infant at birth. These are raised lesions and often do not appear until the infant is a few weeks of age. Deep cavernous hemangiomas are based on the localized failure of normal angiogenesis. They grow slowly after birth and have a blue color because of their site below the dermis. There is a soft movable nonpulsatile mass which feels like a "bag of worms." Blood flow through these tumors is very slow and, therefore, they do not compress easily or blanch with pressure.

1.124

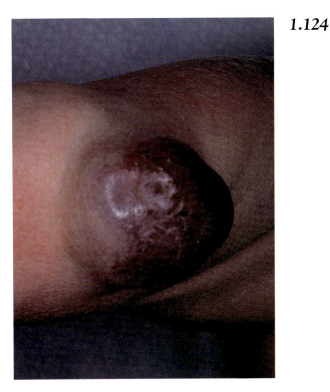

1.125

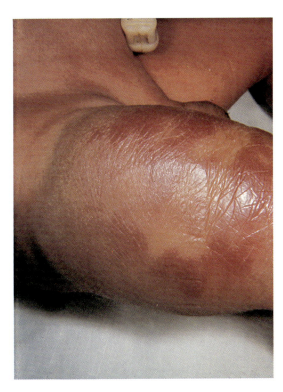

Figure 1.124. Cavernous hemangiomas occur mainly on the head and neck but may present anywhere such as this large cavernous hemangioma of the right knee. Thrombocytopenia due to platelet trapping, and marked vascular shunting leading to high output congestive heart failure may be complications associated with large cavernous hemangiomas.

Figure 1.125. This infant with Kasabach-Merritt syndrome (cavernous hemangioma with thrombocytopenia) had a large cavernous hemangioma of the right lower thigh and knee and a platelet count of 54,000/mm³. These infants may develop disseminated intravascular coagulopathy because of the consumption of the coagulation factors.

1.126

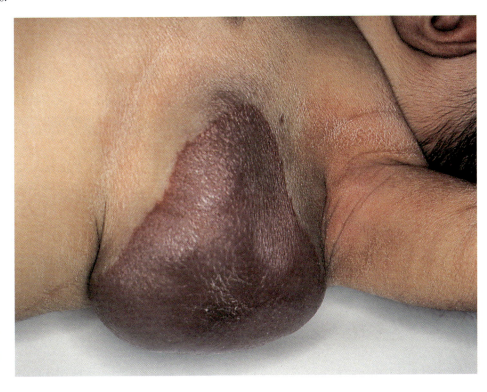

Figure 1.126. This large cavernous hemangioma of the left side of the chest was asymptomatic and the infant had a normal platelet count.

1.127

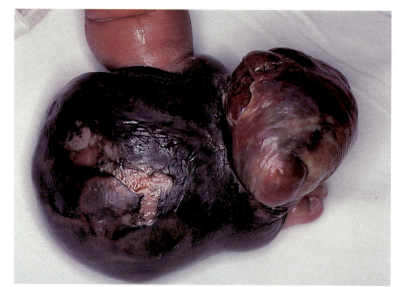

Figure 1.127. The massive cavernous hemangioma involving the left leg and foot of this infant was compromised during in utero life, resulting in gangrene. The hemangioma was removed surgically after birth. In large cavernous hemangiomas the underlying structures may be involved, such as in this infant where the underlying osseous structures were involved.

1.128

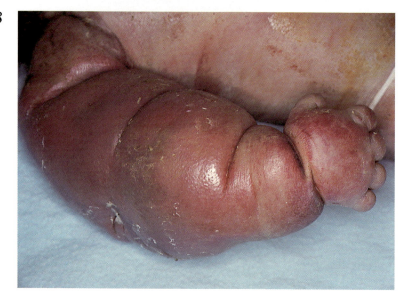

Figure 1.128. The massive cavernous hemangioma of the right upper extremity in this infant resulted in high output congestive heart failure in utero. There was marked anasarca with a total protein of 2.8 mg/dL, hematocrit of 20%, and platelet count of 26,000/mm³.

1.129

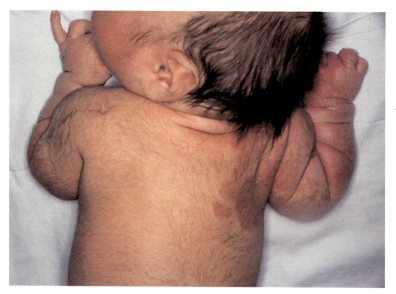

Figure 1.129. A large capillary hemangioma (nevus flammeus) involving the right shoulder and right upper extremity resulting in an asymmetric hypertrophy of the shoulder and right upper extremity. This constitutes the Klippel-Trenaunay syndrome. Unilateral distribution predominates and there may be disproportionate growth. Hypertrophy is not always present at the site of the vascular malformation. The cause of the hemihypertrophy is not definitely known, but it is suggested that it may be due to a local increased blood supply to the area.

1.130

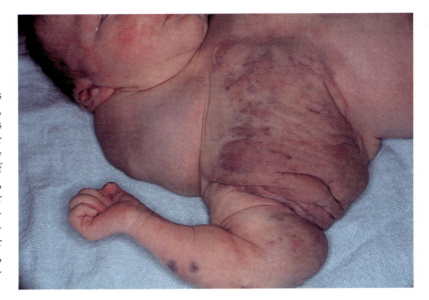

Figure 1.130. The large cavernous hemangioma involving the neck, chest, and axilla of this infant was associated with numerous other small hemangiomas over the body and resulted in hemihypertrophy of the right upper arm, the right leg, and the left foot. This is another example of Klippel-Trenaunay syndrome. In Klippel-Trenaunay syndrome one should always check for hemangiomata of the viscera, brain, and eyes in addition to the involvement of the skin.

1.131

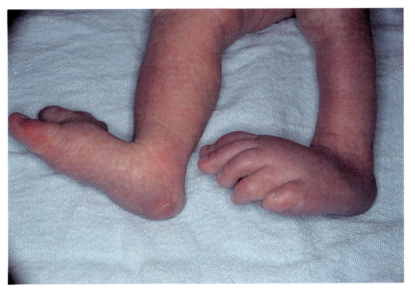

Figure 1.131. The lower extremities of the same infant as in Figure 1.130 with Klippel-Trenaunay syndrome shows the hypertrophy of the right leg and the left foot.

1.132

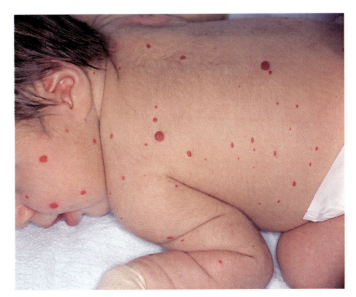

Figure 1.132. Multiple hemangiomatosis (diffuse neonatal hemangiomatosis) may present solely with cutaneous involvement, as noted in this infant, or with systemic involvement (of the liver, brain, etc.). There are numerous widely disseminated, small, red to dark blue papular cutaneous hemangiomas which are usually present at birth or develop within the first few weeks of life. In infants with cutaneous involvement only, prognosis is good. In infants with systemic involvement, prognosis is variable.

1.133

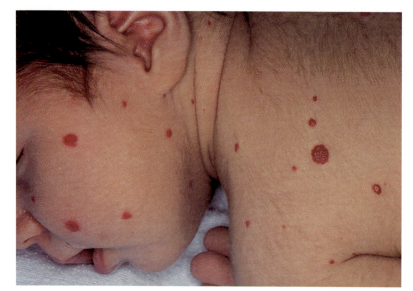

Figure 1.133. A close-up view of the multiple hemangiomata in the same infant as in Figure 1.132.

1.134

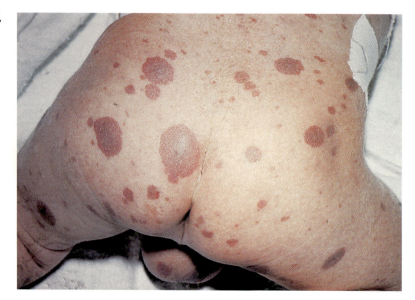

Figure 1.134. Multiple hemangiomatosis in an infant with systemic involvement. There were multiple hemangiomata in the liver and several hemangiomata in the gastrointestinal tract and brain in this infant. At the age of ten days the infant developed hematemesis and abdominal distention. At surgery it was noted the infant had massive hemorrhage from a hemangioma in the duodenum. If systemic involvement is suspected, liver and spleen scans or hepatic angiography may confirm the diagnosis. (See Figure 2.147 of Volume V for an example of systemic involvement in multiple hemangiomatosis.)

1.135

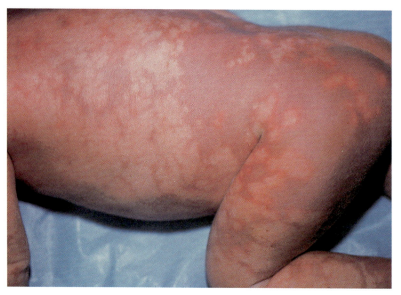

Figure 1.135. In cutis marmorata telangiectatica congenita (congenital generalized lymphangiectasia), dilated superficial venous and capillary channels are usually noted at birth. The skin appears as a reticulated network with white insulae in between. The classic appearance of reddish-blue reticulation of the skin changes with crying (becomes increasingly red) or other stimulation (becomes livid with cooling). Most cases are generalized, such as in this infant, but there may be segmental or localized involvement.

1.136

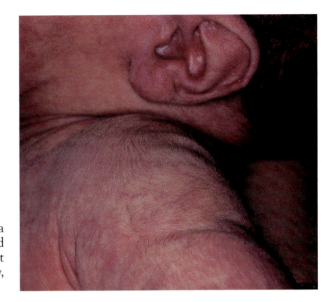

Figure 1.136. Another infant with cutis marmorata telangiectatica congenita. The condition may extend for the first few weeks and usually persists throughout life, but eventually improves during childhood. Rarely, small areas of superficial ulceration may develop.

1.137

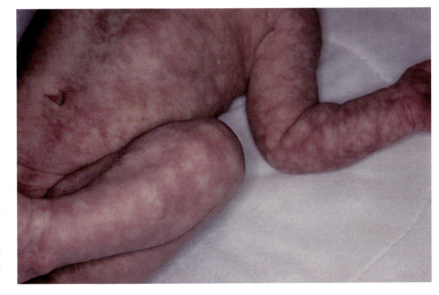

Figure 1.137. Cutis marmorata telangiectatica congenita in which the distribution is segmental. The etiology is unknown, but it seems to represent a developmental ectasia of both capillaries and veins.

1.138

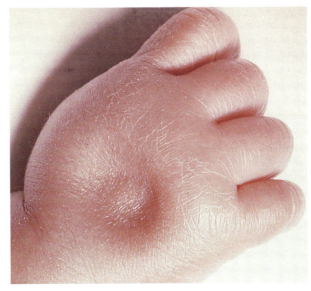

Figure 1.138. Lymphedema in an infant with Turner's syndrome shows pitting edema on the dorsum of the hand. The diffuse soft tissue swelling in lymphedema is caused by increased accumulation of lymph due to inadequate lymphatic drainage. Lymphedema may be primary (congenital) or secondary.

1.139

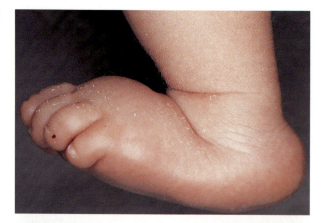

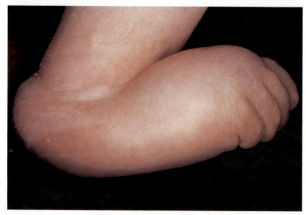

Figure 1.139. Lymphedema of both feet in an infant with Turner's syndrome. The area is swollen and firm at birth and is characterized by pitting on pressure.

1.140

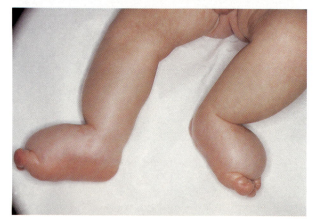

Figure 1.140. Milroy's disease is an inherited autosomal dominant condition which presents with the typical bilateral lymphedema in the lower extremities. The condition occurs as a result of absence of lymphatics and is always confined to the legs and feet.

1.141

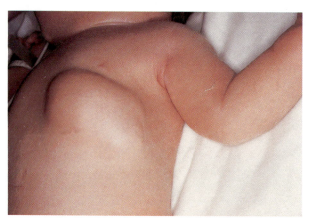

Figure 1.141. Lymphangioma simplex of the anterior chest present at birth in an infant. There are four major forms of lymphangiomas: lymphangioma simplex, lymphangioma circumscriptum, cavernous lymphangioma, and cystic hygroma. Lymphangioma simplex is a solitary, well-circumscribed, flesh-colored dermal or subcutaneous tumor. It may occur anywhere on the subcutaneous or mucosal surface and is seen most commonly on the neck, upper trunk, proximal extremities and tongue. The surface is generally smooth and it may remain stable or grow quickly.

1.142

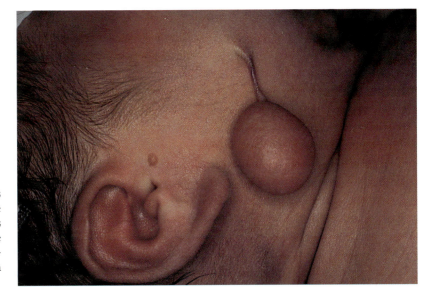

Figure 1.142. On removal, this mass attached by a stalk to the right side of this infant's face was confirmed to be a typical simple lymphangioma. The small preauricular tag was not associated with any other pathology.

1.143

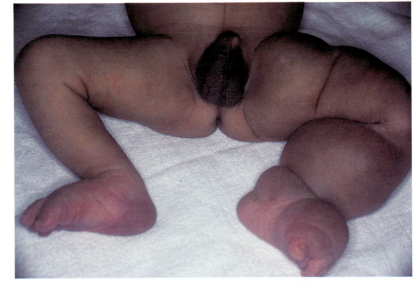

Figure 1.143. Circumscribed lymphangioma of the left lower extremity in a neonate. Lymphangioma circumscriptum is the most common form of lymphangioma. It is characterized by groups of deep-seated, thick-walled vesicles that have the appearance of "frog spawn" or "grape clusters." The common sites of involvement are the proximal limbs, shoulders, neck, axilla and adjacent chest wall, perineum, inguinal folds, tongue, and mucous membranes.

Figure 1.144. A large cavernous lymphangioma of the left axilla and anterior chest present at birth in an infant. Cavernous lymphangioma consists of diffuse soft tissue masses of large cystic dilatations of lymphatic vessels in the dermis and subcutaneous tissue, and may involve the intermuscular septa. The lesions are ill-defined and frequently involve large areas of the face, trunk, and extremities. They may occur in the tongue, resulting in macroglossia. Lymphangiomas frequently have a hemangiomatous component (hemangiolymphoma) so that some of the vesicles are filled with fresh or altered blood. Treatment is surgical but recurrences are common.

1.144

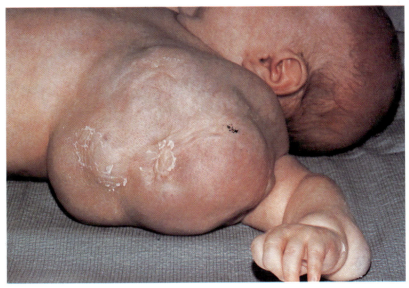

1.145

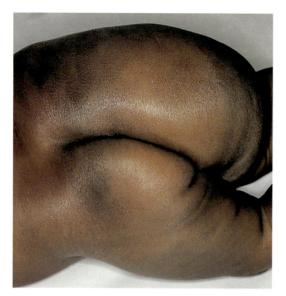

Figure 1.145. A large cavernous lymphangioma affecting the right gluteal region and proximal lower extremity of an infant. There was no osseous involvement.

1.146

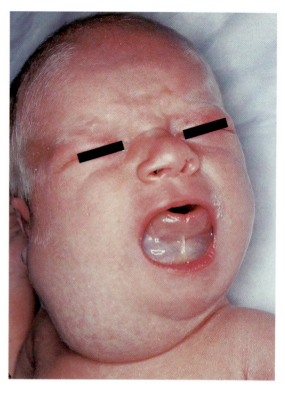

Figure 1.146. Cystic hygroma of the right side of the neck with involvement of the mucous membranes. Cystic hygroma is a benign loculated cystic mass which is soft, diffuse, impressible, and translucent due to accumulation of fluid in the lymphatics. The commonest sites are in the neck (hygroma colli), axilla, and upper arm. Rarely they are seen in the groin or popliteal fossa. They do not resolve spontaneously. Surgical treatment may be complicated and recurrences are uncommon following complete removal.

1.147

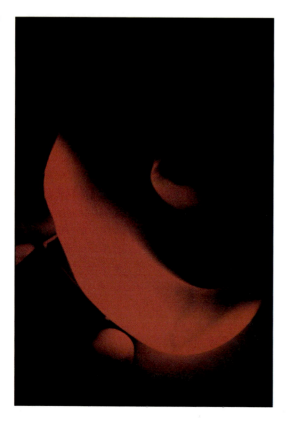

Figure 1.147. Transillumination of the cystic hygroma in the same infant as in Figure 1.146. Note the extent of involvement of the neck and mouth.

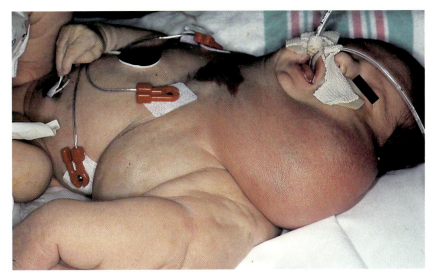

1.148

Figure 1.148. This infant with a massive diffuse lymphangioma (elephantiasis congenita angiomatosis or elephantiasis lymphangiectatica) had severely compromised respiration from the tumor and required tracheostomy. Note the large area of nevus present superficially over the anterior part of the chest. Biopsy diagnosis was a hemangiolymphoma. Note the redness of the area which was related to secondary infection, a common complication.

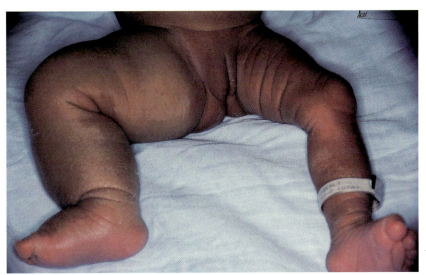

1.149

Figure 1.149. In another infant with elephantiasis congenita angiomatosis, note the massive involvement of the right lower extremity. Diffuse angiomas (elephantiasis lymphangiectatica) are large, ill-defined cystic dilatations involving the skin, subcutaneous tissue, muscles, and mucous membrane. They may involve the trunk, extremities, and large areas of the face, lips, or tongue. There is marked enlargement of the affected areas as a result of invasion by the cystic lymphatics. The areas may have a red or purplish color because of the presence in the vesicles of blood mixed with lymph.

PIGMENTATION ABNORMALITIES

Vitiligo (leukoderma) is a condition which is not commonly seen in the neonatal period. The irregularly outlined hypopigmented areas seen in vitiligo often have hyperpigmented borders, and the patches may enlarge over a period of several years but *will not darken over time*. When areas of hypopigmentation are noted they must be differentiated from the ash leaf appearance of tuberous sclerosis.

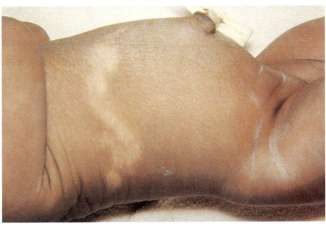

1.150

Figure 1.150. There may be iatrogenic causes of delayed pigmentation, such as a hypopigmented area over the skin where chest electrodes or tape have been placed. These hypopigmented areas occurring as a result of irritation or breakdown of the skin *darken with increasing age* and blend with the surrounding skin.

1.151

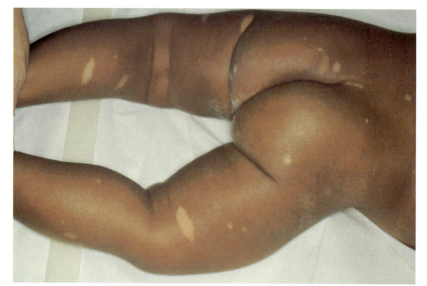

Figure 1.151. Ash leaf spots are found on the skin of the trunk, buttocks, and limbs in children with tuberous sclerosis. These dull, white areas may be linear or oval, measuring 1 cm across or less. They tend to be sharply pointed at one end and rounded at the other. Café-au-lait spots may be present. Ash leaf spots lack the characteristic milky-white appearance of lesions of vitiligo because melanocytes are present in fair numbers but the melanosomes are poorly pigmented.

1.152

Figure 1.152. Examination of the lesions under the Wood's filter shows the typical ash leaf spots in the same infant with tuberous sclerosis. Tuberous sclerosis is a neurocutaneous syndrome which, in addition to the cutaneous changes, has systemic manifestations in 80 to 90% of cases. These include central nervous system involvement (seizures, mental retardation), cardiac tumors (rhabdomyomas), renal hamartomas, retinal lesions, and osseous changes. CT scan may show tumor-like nodes in the cerebral cortex.

1.153

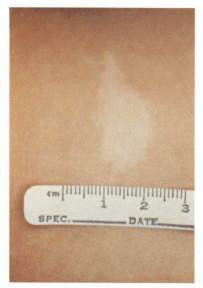

Figure 1.153. A close-up of a typical ash leaf macule in tuberous sclerosis showing the characteristic hypopigmented leaf shape. In tuberous sclerosis, shagreen patches are also noted; these are zones of slightly thickened and firm, yellow, irregularly outlined skin, a few centimeters across, with a finely dimpled surface resembling the skin of an orange. They are usually found on the flanks and back.

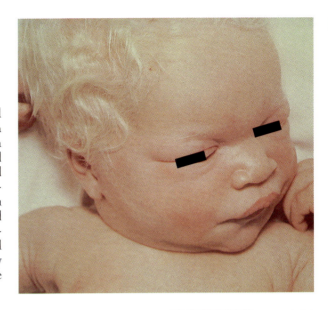

1.154

Figure 1.154. This is a black infant with total albinism, an autosomal recessive condition in which total lack of pigment is characteristic. Albinism is an uncommon disorder of melanin synthesis manifested by a total lack of pigmentation of the skin, hair, and eyes. It occurs in two forms: oculocutaneous and ocular. In oculocutaneous albinism there is generally a decrease or absence of pigment in the eyes, skin, and hair; in ocular albinism only the eye pigment is consistently abnormal. If the iris does not have the typical pink appearance seen in albinism but has a bluish-grey pigmentation, it is less likely that the child will be photophobic.

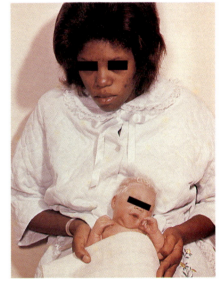

1.155

Figure 1.155. Another infant with albinism with her mother. Note the striking difference in pigmentation of mother and baby. Albinism is characterized by varying degrees of reduction of pigment in the skin and hair, translucent irides, hypopigmented ocular fundi and an associated nystagmus. Affected children have been called "moon children" because they have marked photosensitivity and photophobia, and prefer to go outdoors only at night.

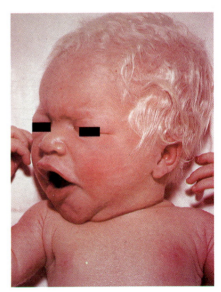

1.156

Figure 1.156. Close-up of the same infant as in Figure 1.154 showing the total lack of pigmentation.

1.157

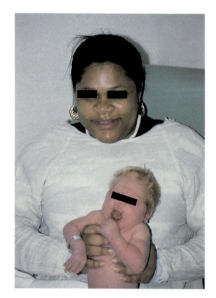

Figure 1.157. Mother and infant with tyrosinase-positive oculocutaneous albinism. Melanocytes or melanosomes are present in the affected skin and hair in normal numbers but, although they are tyrosine positive, fail to produce normal amounts of melanin in the areas of leukoderma or poliosis. There are many variants of oculocutaneous albinism but tyrosinase-positive or tyrosinase-negative are the most common. These are so designated on the basis of pigment production in plucked hair incubated in tyrosine.

1.158

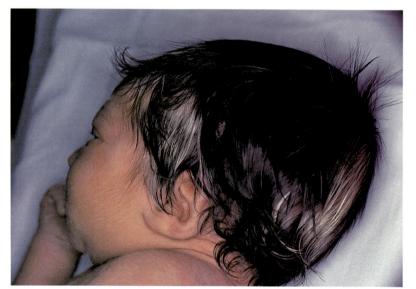

Figure 1.158. In partial albinism (poliosis circumscripta; piebaldism) there are hypopigmented areas of the scalp. Depigmented areas may also occur on the torso or the extremities with the exception of the back, hands, and feet. Decreased hair pigmentation (poliosis) is most often seen close to the anterior hairline either centrally or to one side of the midline. This condition (piebaldism) is seen in normal individuals and may follow an autosomal dominant inheritance.

1.159

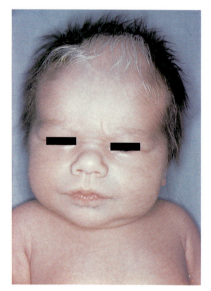

Figure 1.159. In Waardenburg's syndrome, an autosomal dominant condition, a white forelock is characteristic. It is a form of partial albinism (poliosis). In addition to the white forelock, there is dystopia canthorum (lateral displacement of the medial canthi and lacrimal puncta of the lower eyelids), synophrys, heterochromia iridis, broad nasal root, and congenital deafness. If the inner canthal distance divided by the interpupillary distance is greater than 0.6, this lateral displacement of the inner canthi may help confirm the diagnosis.

1.160

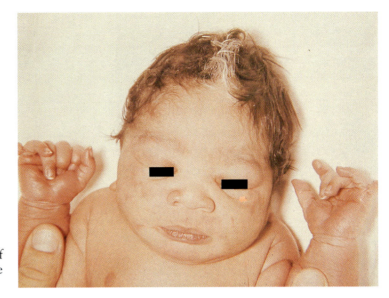

Figure 1.160. Another example of Waardenburg's syndrome. Note the white forelock and the dystopia canthorum.

Figure 1.161. Café-au-lait spots, present in this twin infant with neurofibromatosis, are skin lesions caused by hyperpigmentation of the basal epidermal cells. They may be seen in healthy children, as well as those with neurofibromatosis, tuberous sclerosis, and the Russell-Silver syndrome. They range in size from a few millimeters to several centimeters in diameter and have a color slightly darker than that of the surrounding skin. The most common type have edges that are fairly smooth and quite clearly demarcated ("coast of California"). A second type of café-au-lait spot has a much more jagged, irregular border ("coast of Maine") and is usually larger and solitary. Such lesions are seen in McCune-Albright polyostotic dysplasia.

1.161

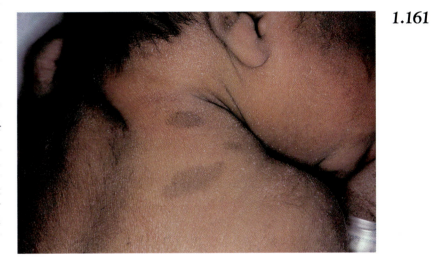

1.162

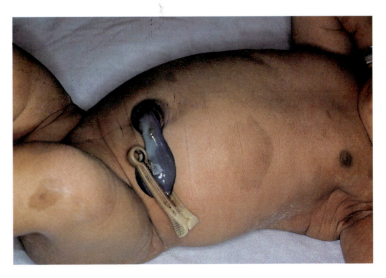

Figure 1.162. In this infant with neurofibromatosis note the multiple café-au-lait spots. About 5% of white infants and almost 15% of black infants have one such spot. Café-au-lait spots are somewhat darker in color in black infants than in caucasian infants. Neurofibromatosis is an autosomal dominant condition in which the presence of 5 or more café-au-lait spots greater than 0.5 cm in diameter in young infants is diagnostic of the disorder.

1.163

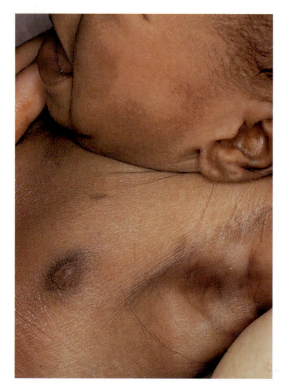

Figure 1.163. Another infant with neurofibromatosis. The presence of a single café-au-lait spot in the axilla may be diagnostic of this disorder. Crowe's sign (axillary freckling) appears as multiple 1- to 4-mm café-au-lait spots in the axillary vault and is seen in 25 to 50% of patients with neurofibromatosis.

1.164

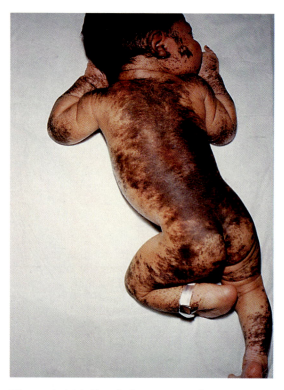

Figure 1.164. Familial progressive hyperpigmentation in a neonate is a benign form of familial hyperpigmentation that has been reported only in black families. The mother was affected and, including this infant, she had five affected children. This dominantly inherited condition presents at birth as irregular patches and streaks of hyperpigmentation which increase in size, number, and confluence with age. The pigmentation later appears in the conjunctivae and buccal mucosa, and extensive areas of the skin and mucous membranes are involved.

1.165

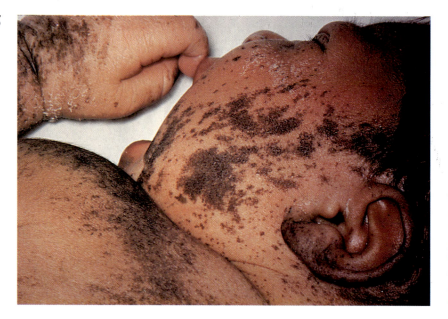

Figure 1.165. A close-up of the face of the same infant as in Figure 1.164 with familial progressive hyperpigmentation. Histopathologically the most distinctive manifestation consists of heavy melanization of the basal cell layers.

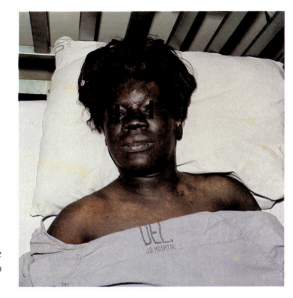

1.166

Figure 1.166. Note the marked hyperpigmentation in the skin of the mother of the infant shown in Fig. 1.165. Also note the pigmentation in the conjunctivae.

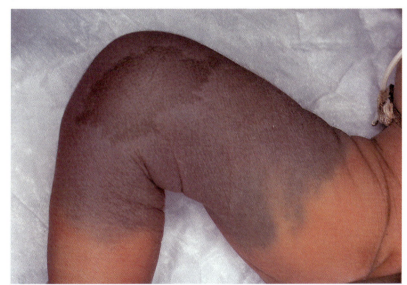

1.167

Figure 1.167. A pigmented nevus (junctional nevus) is a flat melanocytic nevus. The lesions are superficial, flat, discrete, brown, and hyperpigmented. There are usually a few lesions and they have a sharply demarcated border. Their color may vary from brown to black and they are caused by excessive numbers of melanocytes (nevocytes) at the dermal-epidermal junction. In some instances, proliferation of nevocytes down into the dermis occurs, giving rise to a raised, more or less darkly pigmented papular or verrucous lesion. These nevi are usually benign and the potential for malignant change is minimal but is greater for lesions that appear after birth.

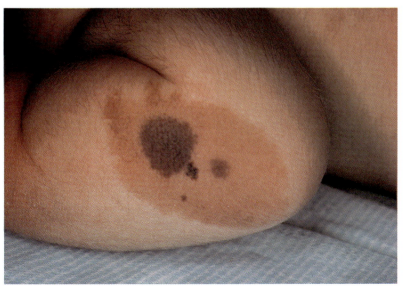

1.168

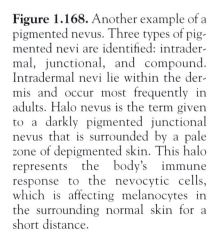

Figure 1.168. Another example of a pigmented nevus. Three types of pigmented nevi are identified: intradermal, junctional, and compound. Intradermal nevi lie within the dermis and occur most frequently in adults. Halo nevus is the term given to a darkly pigmented junctional nevus that is surrounded by a pale zone of depigmented skin. This halo represents the body's immune response to the nevocytic cells, which is affecting melanocytes in the surrounding normal skin for a short distance.

1.169

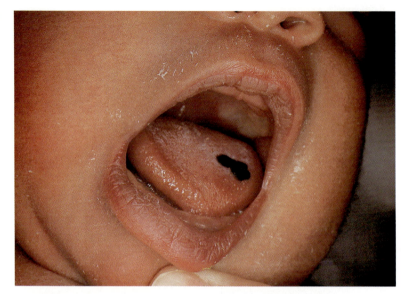

Figure 1.169. The pigmented nevus of the tongue is another example of a junctional nevus in an unusual location.

1.170

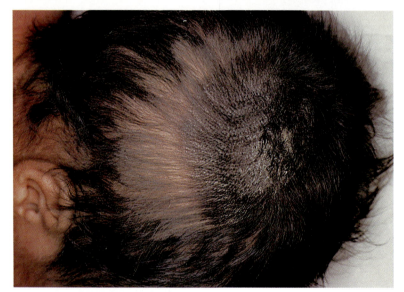

Figure 1.170. A pigmented nevus on the scalp obviously has associated hair and, because of this, tends to be much coarser in texture. These junctional nevi of the scalp may cover large areas.

1.171

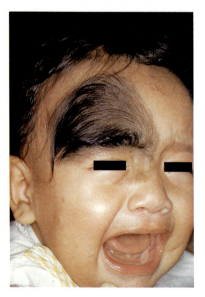

Figure 1.171. In this infant there is a large benign hairy pigmented nevus. These nevi may be pale at first with fine vellus hairs, but increasing pigmentation takes place during the first year of life, often with the growth of dark coarse hair. The hyperpigmented zones may be extremely large with numerous satellite lesions. They may occur anywhere on the body and are variable in size. Approximately 10% of giant hairy nevi develop into malignant melanomas.

Figure 1.172. A congenital giant pigmented nevus is extensive and sharply outlined. The hyperpigmented zones may be extremely large, covering the trunk, especially the lower trunk ("garment" nevus or "bathing trunk" nevus). "Garment" nevi involve a very large body surface area (e.g., the entire back or an extremity). The surface of these lesions is nodular or raised with fleshy elements and has a somewhat leathery texture. It may have dark, coarse hairs within the lesion. Histologically this would be classified as a compound nevus. A junctional nevus lies only on the epidermal surface and is flat, smooth, and relatively small. Junctional nevi over time may become compound nevi. Compound nevi possess the features of both junctional and intradermal nevi in that nevus cells are seen within the dermis as well as within the epidermis. They tend to be more elevated and vary from a slightly raised plaque to a lesion of a somewhat more papillomatous nature.

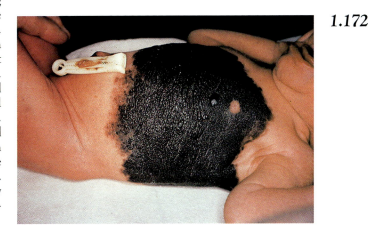

1.172

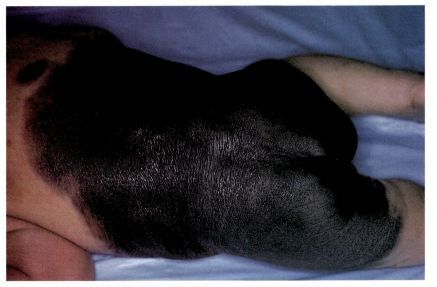

1.173

Figure 1.173. A large "garment" nevus involving most of the trunk and perineum. In infants with a giant "garment" nevus there may be widely disseminated pigmented patches which represent satellite melanocytic nevi. In these infants there is a propensity for malignant change, and therefore an aggressive surgical approach is justified.

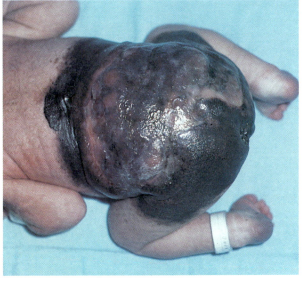

1.174

Figure 1.174. This infant with a large "garment" ("bathing trunk") nevus had skin breakdown with ulceration in utero and presented at birth with this appearance. Examination of the placenta showed numerous secondary pigmented nevi in the placental tissue. Histopathologic examination of the nevi in the placenta showed numerous melanoma cells. The mother was normal.

1.175

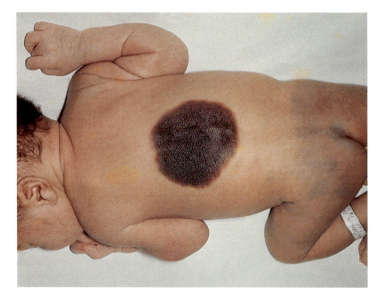

Figure 1.175. A large pigmented nevus over the midline in the thoracolumbar area of this infant may be significant in that any lesion located in the midline over the spine should alert one to the possibility of a neural tube defect. The faun-tail nevus is an elongated patch of dark skin bearing abundant long dark hair located in the midline over the lumbar spine or sacrum. It is a rare but helpful indicator of a tethered spinal cord.

1.176

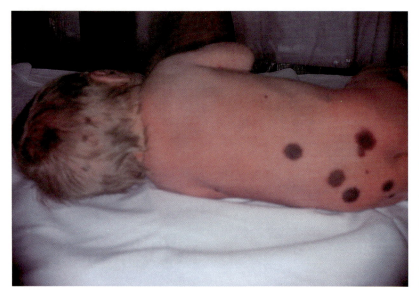

Figure 1.176. The multiple pigmented nevi involving the scalp and trunk in this infant are characteristic of the neurocutaneous melanosis sequence. There are dark pigmented multiple nevi, which are sometimes hairy and are more extensive in a bathing trunk distribution over the lower trunk, abdomen, and lower thighs. There may be leptomeningeal involvement with nests and sheets of melanoblasts, most striking at the base of the brain. This may lead to hydrocephalus, seizures, and deterioration of central nervous system function. In these cases, cells containing melanin may be detected in the cerebrospinal fluid.

1.177

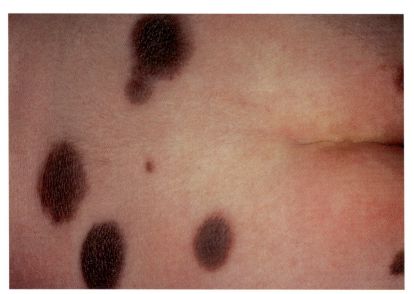

Figure 1.177. A close-up of the lesions in the lumbosacral and gluteal areas in the same infant as in Figure 1.176.

1.178

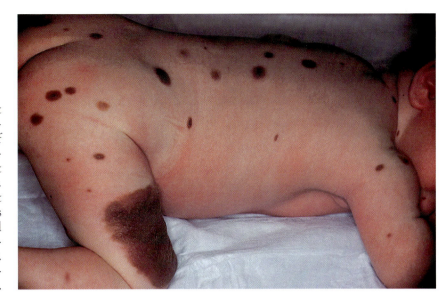

Figure 1.178. Another infant with the neurocutaneous melanosis sequence. The finding of a single giant nevus with numerous satellite lesions is not uncommon in this disorder. Cutaneous melanosis is evident at birth and central nervous system function may be normal initially, but seizures and mental deterioration occur later. The risk of malignant melanoma degeneration is 10 to 15%.

1.179

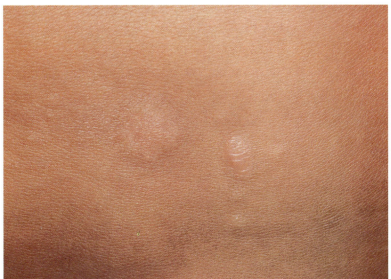

Figure 1.179. Mastocytosis (urticaria pigmentosa) is a mast cell infiltrative disorder which presents at birth or develops during the first few weeks of life. The lesions may be solitary or in groups, as in this infant. Macules, papules, nodular lesions, vesicles, and bullae may all be signs of mastocytosis. They vary in color from a slightly reddish appearance to a tan or brown appearance. Spontaneous remission of the skin lesions usually occurs. Skin biopsy shows mast cell infiltration.

1.180

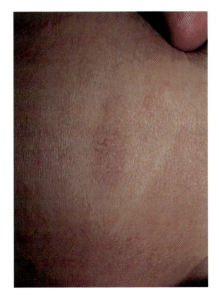
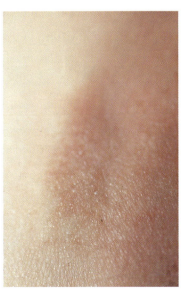

Figure 1.180. In about 5% of cases, mastocytosis is localized. In the figure on the left there is a solitary tan to brownish-colored, slightly raised lesion on the back. As seen in the figure on the right, rubbing the skin over this area results in dermatographism (Darier's sign) due to histamine release. Nodular forms of mastocytosis must be differentiated from xanthoma and juvenile xanthomagranulomas.

1.181

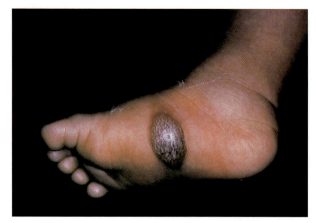

Figure 1.181. This is a lesion of bullous mastocytosis (urticaria pigmentosa) that presented at birth in this infant as a solitary bullous lesion on the sole of the right foot. Note the area of redness surrounding the lesion (dermatographism) following examination of the lesion. Spontaneous remission of the skin lesions usually occurs. It is rare for lesions to appear after the age of 3 years. Differential diagnosis includes bullous impetigo, epidermolysis bullosa, incontinentia pigmenti, and bullous congenital ichthyosiform erythroderma.

1.182

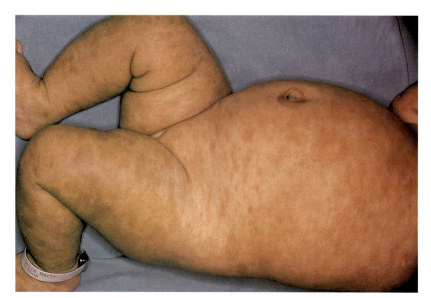

Figure 1.182. In this infant with a systemic skin rash present at birth, the diagnosis of urticaria pigmentosa was confirmed. In systemic mastocytosis there is hepatosplenomegaly and bone involvement. Biopsy shows mast cell infiltration. In localized mastocytosis, which occurs in about 5% of all cases of mastocytosis, spontaneous remission of the skin lesions usually occurs. Prognosis is usually good, provided that there are no signs of systemic mastocytosis (hepatosplenomegaly, bone involvement).

1.183

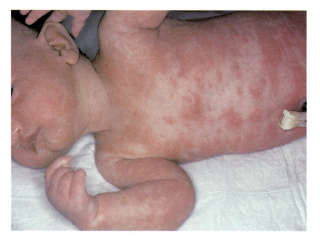

Figure 1.183. Incontinentia pigmenti (Bloch-Sulzberger syndrome) is considered to be a neurocutaneous syndrome seen only in female infants (X-linked dominant, generally lethal prenatally to the male). It has four cutaneous phases. In this infant note the early maculopapular appearance without vesicles or pigmentation. The lesions contain eosinophils, and blood eosinophilia is frequently present. In the next phase there are many vesicular lesions. These then become bullous and pustular. The bullae may be superseded by verrucous lesions in the same distribution, and after these disappear, whorls of hyperpigmentation appear. In the final phase, hypopigmented patches may occur. The patterning of the skin abnormalities follows the path of Blaschko's lines, which represent the course of early migration of primordial skin cells progressing from the dorsal to the ventral midline.

1.184

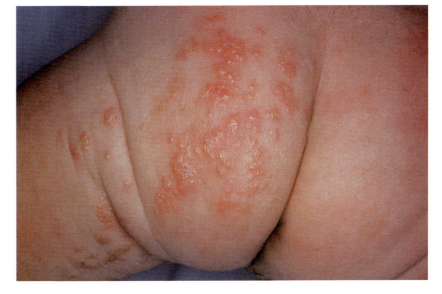

Figure 1.184. Within the first month of life in incontinentia pigmenti, the vesicular phase develops as noted in this infant. Note the linearly arranged vesicles and red nodules on the flexor surface of the upper and lower extremities. The blisters may cluster in a bizarre arrangement if they are numerous.

1.185

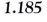
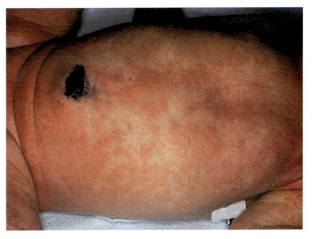

Figure 1.185. Another infant with incontinentia pigmenti. Note the maculovesicular pigmented appearance of the skin in a swirling pattern. The infant developed seizures on the 2nd day of life. Systemic manifestations occur in about 70% of infants (20% at birth). These include central nervous system (microcephaly, seizures, and retardation), ocular (cataracts, retinal dysplasia, etc.), osseous (hemivertebrae, extra ribs, hemiatrophy, etc.), dental (hypodontia, etc.), and occasionally cardiac abnormalities.

1.186

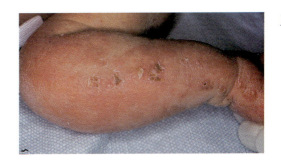

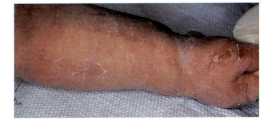

Figure 1.186. In this phase of incontinentia pigmenti, vesicles and bullae have formed and these have broken down with some increased pigmentation.

1.187

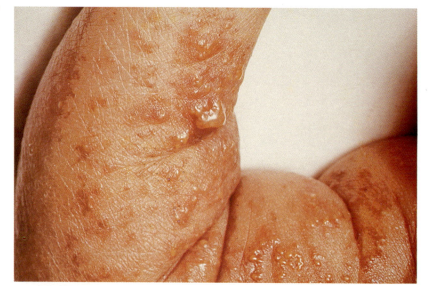

Figure 1.187. A close-up of the right upper extremity showing the vesicles with some verrucous element and increasing pigmentation with a tendency to follow Blaschko's lines.

1.188

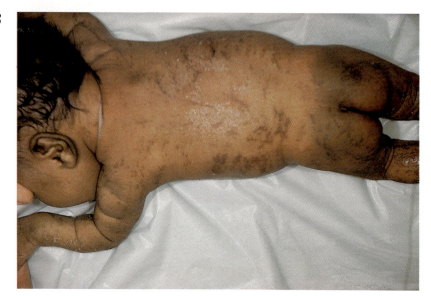

Figure 1.188. In a later phase of incontinentia pigmenti, between 6 to 12 months of age, red-brown, hyperpigmented lesions appear in a symmetric distribution on the arms and legs while other lesions have improved. Note the bizarre distribution of the lesions and the pigmentation. The pigmented zones have very irregular patterns and tend to follow the path of Blaschko's lines. They have a roughly V-shaped configuration over the back, a wavy S-shaped distribution over the anterior trunk, and a longitudinal orientation over the limbs. These lesions tend to persist.

1.189

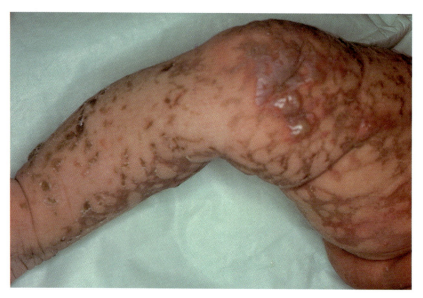

Figure 1.189. A close-up of the right lower extremity of an infant with incontinentia pigmenti. Note the presence of vesicles and the typical pattern of swirled hyperpigmentation of the skin that has been compared to that of a marble cake. This is present mainly on the extremities and trunk, and increases in intensity until the 2nd year of life. It may persist many years, then gradually fades.

1.190

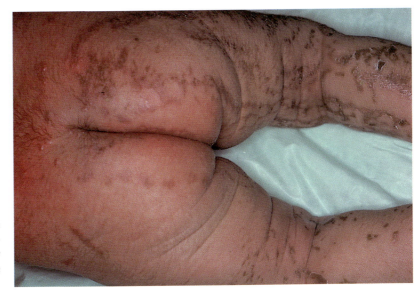

Figure 1.190. A close-up of the lower trunk, buttocks, and extremities showing the pigmentary changes which tend to follow the path of Blaschko's lines.

1.191

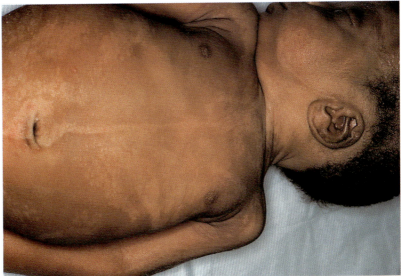

Figure 1.191. In incontinentia pigmenti achromians (hypomelanosis of Ito), a neurocutaneous syndrome, the distribution of hypopigmentation is similar to that of the hyperpigmented areas seen in incontinentia pigmenti. Note that there is a pattern of swirled hypopigmentation which looks like a photographic negative of the hyperpigmented streaks seen in incontinentia pigmenti. This disorder is associated with seizures and mental retardation. The whorls may appear without the prior development of vesicles or bullae.

1.192

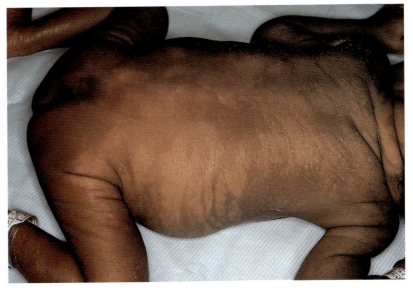

Figure 1.192. The back of the same infant as in Figure 1.191 showing the distribution of the hypopigmented lesions, again demonstrating these bizarre patterns which look like a photographic negative of the hyperpigmented streaks seen in incontinentia pigmenti and which tend to follow Blaschko's lines. In a few patients, the lesions may be patchy and confined to relatively limited areas of the body. In most cases, however, the hypopigmented areas are extensive, often bilateral, and appear to be more pronounced on the ventral surface of the trunk and the flexor surface of the limbs.

1.193

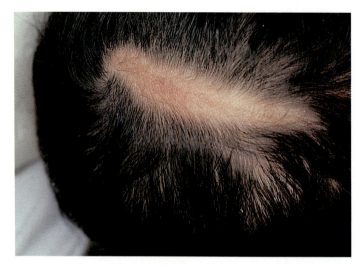

Figure 1.193. Epidermal nevus on the scalp present at birth. These are raised verrucous lesions of variable size, sometimes round but more commonly linear, and tend to follow Blaschko's lines. They may appear later in infancy and are slightly hyperpigmented or yellowish in light-skinned infants, while appearing dark brown to black in darker skinned infants. An epidermal nevus must be differentiated from a nevus sebaceus of Jadassohn.

1.194

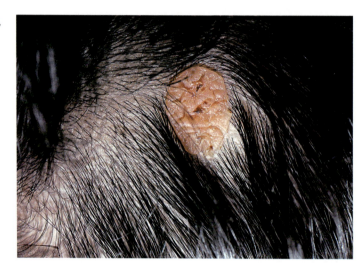

Figure 1.194. Another example of an epidermal nevus on the scalp which was present at birth but had a more verrucous and hyperpigmented appearance. An epidermal nevus is a benign congenital disorder that is characterized by circumscribed hyperkeratosis and hypertrophy of the epidermis. The diagnosis was confirmed by skin biopsy.

1.195

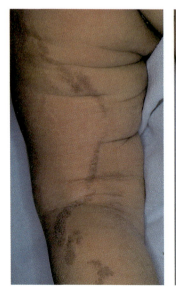 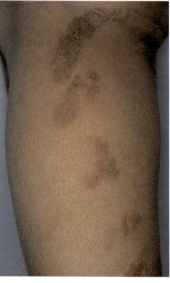

Figure 1.195. A linear epidermal nevus of the back of the left thigh and leg which was present at birth. In this infant note the linearity and the increased pigmentation of the lesions on the thigh. Epidermal nevi often favor the extremities rather than the head and neck in what appears to be a dermatomal distribution (follows Blaschko's lines). They may occur as single lesions, but generally multiple lesions are present arranged in a linear distribution.

1.196

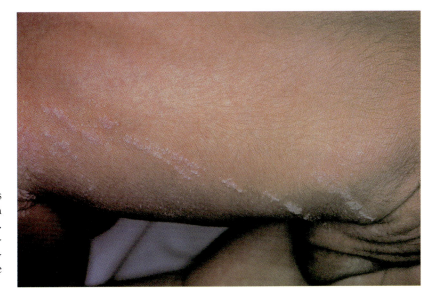

Figure 1.196. Linear verrucous epidermal nevus present at birth over the right torso of an infant. Note that this is similar to an epidermal nevus but has a more verrucous appearance and may be more hyperpigmented.

1.197

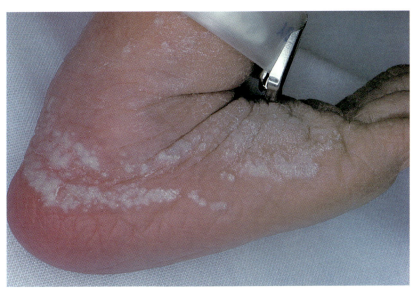

Figure 1.197. Close-up of a linear verrucous epidermal nevus which was present only on the distal part of the left leg and foot of this otherwise normal infant. A localized form (nevus verrucosus) usually consists of a solitary lesion which may be grayish to yellowish-brown in color and warty, granular, or papillomatous in appearance.

1.198

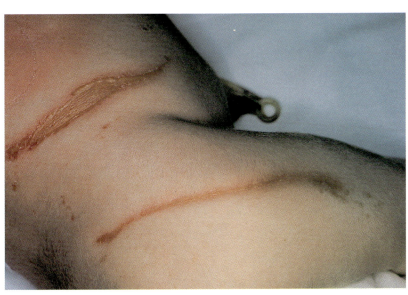

Figure 1.198. This infant presented at birth with linear erosions which were open and appeared to be traumatic. By the age of three months the erosions became hypertrophic and hyperkeratotic. New areas developed over the previous uninvolved areas of the skin, and later a verrucous appearance developed. Skin biopsy diagnosis was that of a classic linear verrucous epidermal nevus. Central nervous system, ocular, and long bone studies were normal.

1.199

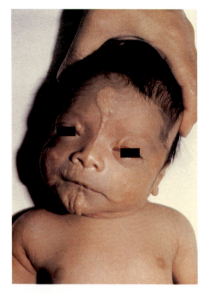

Figure 1.199. Nevus unius lateris is the term used when the lesions of epidermal nevus are extensive and systematized. It may present as a single linear or spiral warty lesion or, at times, as an elaborate, continuous, or interrupted pattern affecting multiple sites. When the scalp, face, or neck is involved, adnexal tissues such as the sebaceous glands may be affected and become enlarged. For this form, the term linear nevus sebaceus may be used. Linear nevus sebaceus should not be confused with nevus sebaceus of Jadassohn, a distinct and unrelated disorder.

In the linear nevus sebaceus syndrome, small linearly arranged verrucous yellow-orange nodules are seen on the face, neck, and limbs. Multiple sebaceous nevi may be found on the scalp and there may be pigmented nevi on the extremities. These lesions may be associated with ocular dermoids and major ophthalmic abnormalities (cloudy cornea and colobomata of the eyelid, iris, and/or choroid). In the central nervous system there may be intracranial malformations which are associated with seizure disorders. Pigmentary and skeletal abnormalities may also be present.

1.200

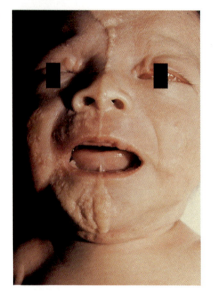

Figure 1.200. Close-up of the face of the same infant as in Figure 1.199 with the linear nevus sebaceus syndrome. Note the typical lesions in the midfacial area which extend from the forehead down into the lower jaw. Note that these are linear in distribution. Also note the dermoids of the eye. This infant developed seizures at the age of 10 days. The EEG was grossly abnormal and a diagnosis of cortical atrophy was made. The infant died at the age of 2 months.

1.201

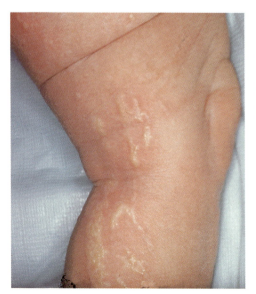
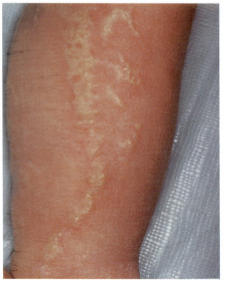

Figure 1.201. Linear epidermal nevi in another infant who had central nervous system abnormalities and seizures.

1.202

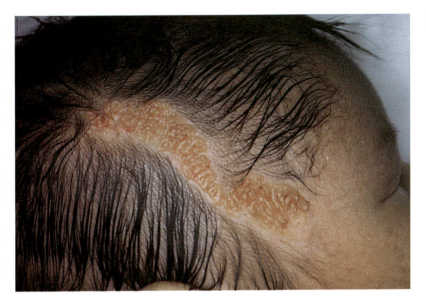

Figure 1.202. Nevus sebaceus of Jadassohn is a hamartomatous lesion with mixed tissue components that most commonly occurs on the scalp and face. These nevi are seen at birth as flat or slightly elevated, well-circumscribed, sometimes elongated, orange-yellow to yellowish-brown plaques with a greasy or waxy hairless surface. The lesions are usually solitary, round or oval on the scalp, or linear on the face and ears. They vary from a few millimeters to centimeters in diameter. The condition is not inherited but familial forms may occur, are noted with equal frequency in males and females, and occur in all races.

1.203

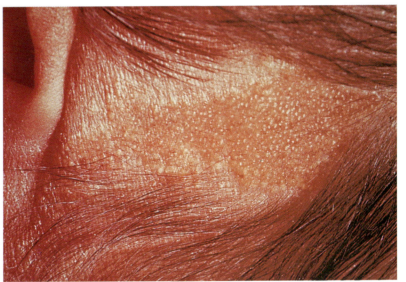

Figure 1.203. Another example of a nevus sebaceus of Jadassohn. Note that this lesion is larger and not as raised as the nevus in the previous infant. The lesions persist, enlarge gradually, and malignant degeneration may occur in 10 to 15% of lesions generally during adolescence or adult life. The most frequent change is that of a basal cell carcinoma. Rapid enlargement or ulceration of the nevus at any age may suggest malignant change.

1.204

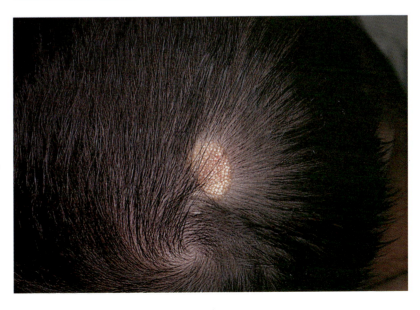

Figure 1.204. Nevus sebaceus of Jadassohn in the scalp. Note that this is a round, small lesion which could easily be missed on the initial physical examination. Linear epidermal nevi and verrucous nevi should not be confused with nevus sebaceus of Jadassohn which is a distinct and unrelated disorder.

1.205

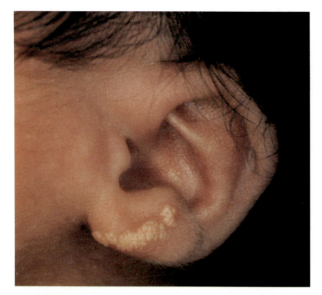

Figure 1.205. An example of a nevus sebaceus of Jadassohn involving the left ear.

1.206

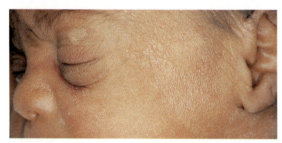

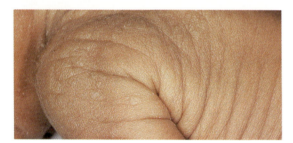

Figure 1.206. Note the raised lesions on the face (upper figure) and similar lesions on the left shoulder and back (lower figure) present at birth in this infant who was otherwise normal. Skin biopsy diagnosis was that of nevoid, unclassified. This is a benign hamartomatous nevus in which the skin lesions are of different cell types and vary considerably in size and location.

VESICULOBULLOUS ERUPTIONS

1.207

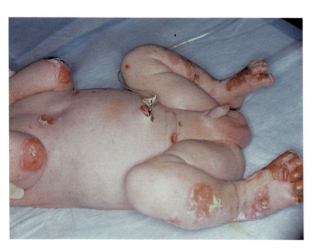

Figure 1.207. Epidermolysis bullosa is an autosomally inherited blistering and bullous disorder which is present at birth or becomes manifest soon after birth. It commonly affects the face, hands, feet, and variably the limbs and trunk and is characterized by trauma-inflicted erosions (Nikolsky's sign) and loss of the epidermis. As in this infant, the lesions are most commonly seen over the extensor surfaces and there are broken bullae with underlying erythroderma. Epidermolysis bullosa occurs in three major inherited forms: e. bullosa simplex (epidermolytic), junctional e. bullosa (letalis; gravis), and e. bullosa dystrophica (dominant and recessive forms) based on the presence or absence of scarring, the mode of inheritance, and the level of skin cleavage following minor trauma.

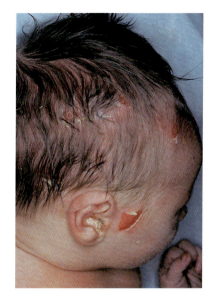

1.208

Figure 1.208. In this infant with epidermolysis bullosa, pressure of the forceps blade at delivery has resulted in a positive Nikolsky's sign. In Nikolsky's sign, firm stroking or rubbing of the skin will cause development of localized separation and tearing of the skin. In the Koebner phenomenon, minimal trauma (rubbing of the skin) may result in the formation of blebs (vesicles and bullae). Vesicles are blistering lesions less than 0.5 cm in diameter, whereas bullae are blistering lesions 0.5 to 1 cm or more in diameter.

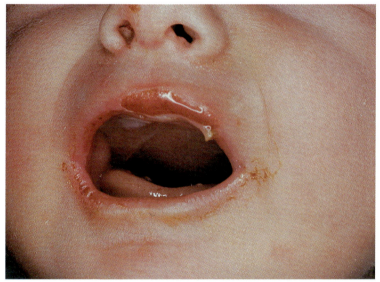

1.209

Figure 1.209. Bullous formation on the lip of the same infant as in Figure 1.208 as a result of resuscitation.

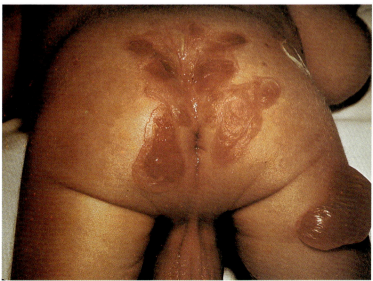

1.210

Figure 1.210. In epidermolysis bullosa simplex, an autosomal dominant condition, there is inadequate bonding between the epidermal and dermal layers with separation of the skin at the basal cell and intraepidermal junction. When the bullae break, the denuded areas resemble second degree burns but the ulcerated vesicles and bullae resolve without scarring and heal rapidly. (Sometimes in severe cases there may be mild scarring.) Mucous membranes and nails are usually not affected.

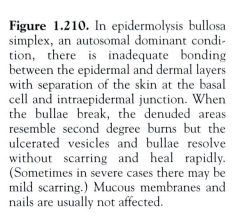

1.211

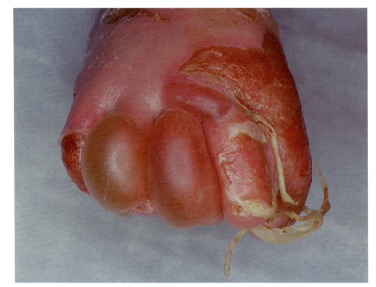

Figure 1.211. Note the bullae on the third and fourth toes and the extensive erosions (after rupture of the bullae) elsewhere on the foot of this infant with the dystrophic form of epidermolysis bullosa. In dystrophic epidermolysis bullosa, the blister forms in the papillary dermis below the basement membrane. These areas heal gradually, leaving atrophic scars, keloids, and contractures. Fingers and toes are bound together if there is loss of digits, and a mitten-like mass may form. Dystrophy of the nails may occur, leading to loss of the nails. This is an autosomal recessive condition which affects skin, mucous membranes and nails.

1.212

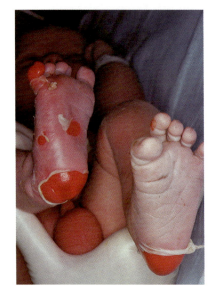

Figure 1.212. Epidermolysis bullosa in which the lesions were present at birth. The feet are one of the most commonly affected sites because babies kick their feet. If the lesions are extensive, the infant is at risk for fluid and electrolyte loss as well as infection.

Figure 1.213. Epidermolysis bullosa letalis (junctional epidermolysis bullosa, Herlitz's disease) in an infant with generalized involvement of the skin. Note the massive involvement of the lower extremities showing the denudation, scarring, and contractures. In this form of epidermolysis bullosa, the skin separates in the lamina lucida of the dermal-epidermal junction and blistering leads to mild atrophic changes. Junctional epidermolysis bullosa is the most severe form of epidermolysis bullosa. It is characterized by blistering and large erosions, mainly on the buttocks, trunk, and scalp without scarring unless complicated by secondary infection. Approximately 50% of these infants die within the first 2 years of life; some survive into adulthood. Therefore, recently the term "letalis" has not been used.

1.213

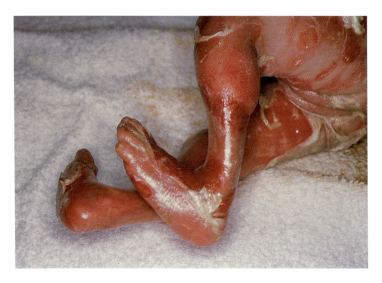

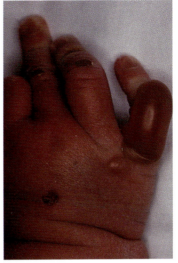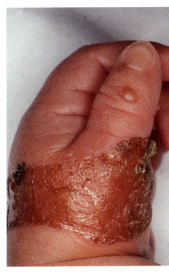

1.214

Figure 1.214. In transient bullous dermolysis of the newborn, the lesions are present at birth or shortly thereafter. With the bullous appearance of the lesions, epidermolysis bullosa should be considered in the differential diagnosis, but the family history and rapid regression of the lesions can confirm the diagnosis of transient bullous dermolysis of the newborn. The sibling of this infant had similar lesions at birth. In the figure on the left note the large bullous lesions on the 5th finger of the right hand. There were similar lesions on the left hand at birth. In the figure on the right note the healing of the lesions 5 days after birth.

SCALING DISORDERS

Different abnormalities of the stratum corneum are included under the general heading "ichthyosis." These conditions all involve faulty keratinization. The name is derived from the small plates of thickened epidermis yielding a pattern similar to the scales of a fish.

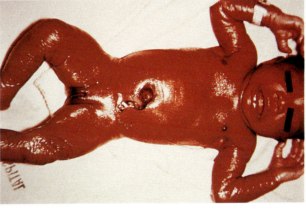

1.215

Figure 1.215. This postmature infant is an example of a so-called "collodion baby." Collodion babies are seen in postmaturity, lamellar ichthyosis, and congenital ichthyosiform erythroderma. The term "collodion" is used because of the varnished (glistening parchment-like) appearance of the skin which is similar to that resulting from collodion applied to the skin. This infant was postmature and the skin improved rapidly.

Figure 1.216. Another example of a collodion baby is this infant with lamellar ichthyosis who was born encased in a membrane. In addition to the collodion appearance of the skin, note the ectropion (eversion of the eyelids with exposure of the palpebral fissure) and eclabium (eversion of the lips which causes inability to suck) which occur as a result of the puckering of the skin, and the hyperkeratosis of the palms and soles. Mobility of the infant may be limited by the tightness of the membrane and also respiratory difficulty may occur due to restriction of chest expansion until spontaneous peeling begins in the first few days. The cutaneous covering dries out and is gradually shed in large sheet-like layers leaving a residual redness and hyperkeratosis.

Lamellar ichthyosis is inherited as an autosomal recessive trait with two variants: the classic, more severe form of lamellar ichthyosis, and a milder erythrodermic variant (non-bullous ichthyosiform erythroderma). (Levy, M., Moise, K.)

1.216

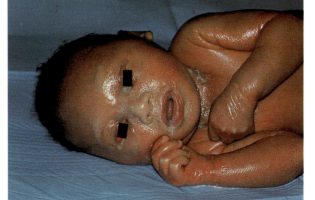

1.217

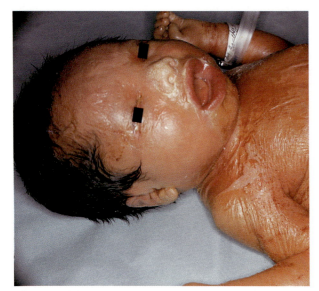

Figure 1.217. Another infant with a milder form of lamellar ichthyosis in which the parchment-like appearance of the skin is not as generalized. The skin develops widespread scaliness which may result in a generalized scaly erythroderma. If scaling and erythroderma are extensive, there may be excessive fluid loss resulting in hypernatremia, dehydration, and temperature instability. These infants are also more susceptible to infection.

1.218

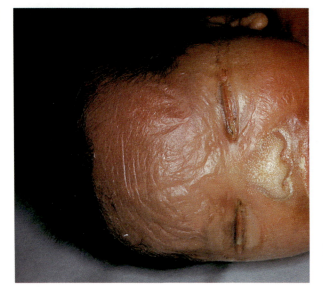

Figure 1.218. Close-up of the face of the same infant as in Figure 1.217, showing the parchment-like appearance of the skin and the mild ectropion.

1.219

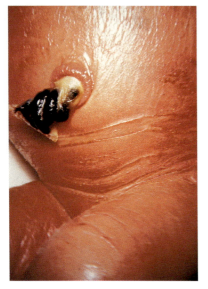

Figure 1.219. Close-up of the abdominal wall and thigh of the same infant as in Figures 1.217 and 1.218 with lamellar ichthyosis. Note the ichthyotic appearance of the skin, particularly in the upper abdomen, and the marked fissuring of the skin below as a result of spontaneous peeling. The underlying skin may be normal or may scale and form a new membrane. Lamellar scales are most prominent over the face, trunk, and extremities. Nail involvement is variable.

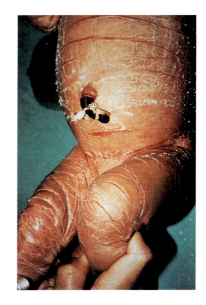

1.220

Figure 1.220. Congenital ichthyosis may present as a hyperkeratotic form in which widespread scaling occurs frequently with underlying erythroderma.

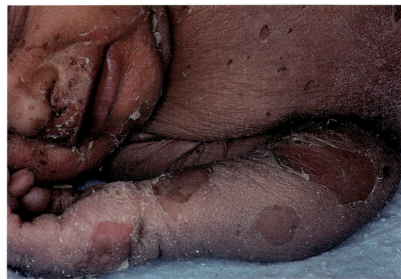

1.221

Figure 1.221. In bullous congenital ichthyosiform erythroderma (epidermolytic hyperkeratosis) there is a combination of bullous lesions, erythema, and desquamation. The presence of bullae is highly characteristic of this disorder. The blisters occur in crops and vary from 0.5 cm to several cm in diameter. They are superficial, tender, and when ruptured leave raw denuded areas. The bullous lesions present at birth and result in the erythema and scaling as noted here. The differential diagnosis includes epidermolysis bullosa, toxic epidermal necrolysis, and the different types of ichthyosis.

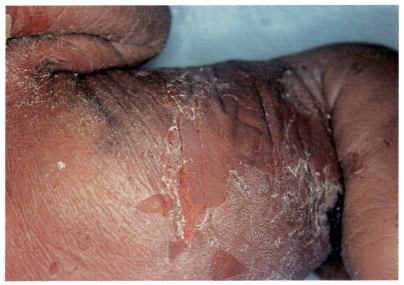

1.222

Figure 1.222. The torso of the same infant as in Figure 1.221 showing the typical erythema and desquamation following rupture of the bullous lesions. Improvement is rapid in these infants and with healing a generalized hyperkeratosis may remain. This consists of thick grayish-brown scales which cover most of the skin surface especially the flexural creases and intertriginous areas which may show marked involvement often with furrowed hyperkeratosis.

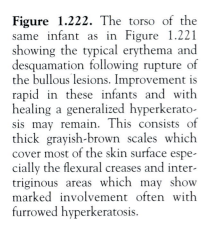

1.223

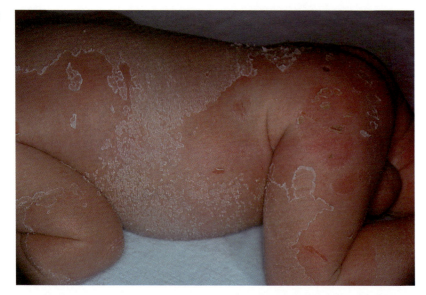

Figure 1.223. Another example of a milder form of the bullous congenital ichthyosiform erythroderma.

1.224

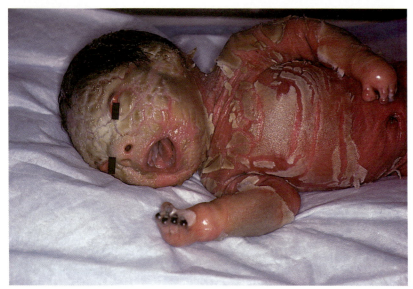

Figure 1.224. Harlequin fetus (congenital ichthyosis) is the most severe form of ichthyosis. It is an autosomal recessive condition which has generally been regarded as being incompatible with life. There is a tight constricting integument with a leather-like consistency. The skin, in addition to being thick and rigid, is cracked and hard with deep crevices. Survival is rare, with death occurring as a result of respiratory insufficiency due to thoracic rigidity, and infection. The harlequin fetus often has unexplained fever and failure to thrive.

1.225

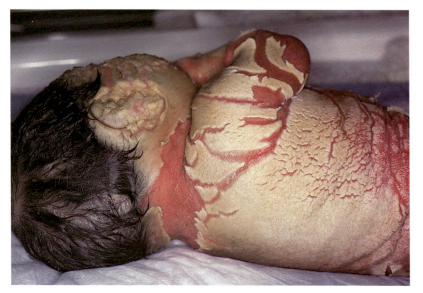

Figure 1.225. Close-up of the head and upper trunk of the same infant as in Figure 1.224. Note the thick, dry, rigid, hardened, cracked skin with deep crevices. The division of the thickened grey- to yellow-colored skin into polygonal, triangular or diamond-shaped plaques by the deep reddish to purple fissures has been said to simulate the traditional costume of a harlequin. The skin has been likened to the bark of a tree, crocodile skin, or Moroccan leather.

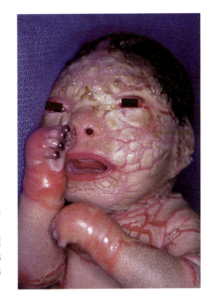

1.226

Figure 1.226. A close-up view of the face and left upper extremity of the same infant as in Figure 1.224 and 1.225. Note the marked ectropion resulting from rigidity of the skin about the eyes with conjunctival redness and edema. There is eclabium with some cracking and fissuring at the corners as a result of the unyielding skin. The right hand is severely affected and has resulted in gangrene of the fingers. The left hand has similar involvement.

1.227

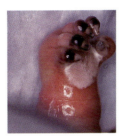 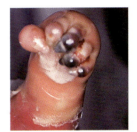

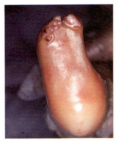 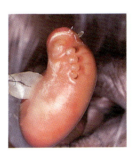

Figure 1.227. The hands and feet of the same harlequin fetus as in Figures 1.224, 1.225 and 1.226 show severe deformities which have occurred as a result of the tight constricting integument and compromise of the ectodermal structures, resulting in gangrene of the fingers and hypoplastic toes. The hands and feet are ischemic, hard, and waxy, often with poorly developed digits and an associated rigid and claw-like appearance of the limbs. The nails may be hypoplastic or absent.

1.228

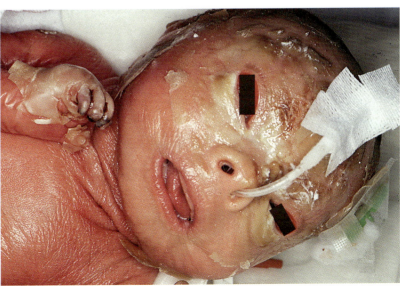

Figure 1.228. Another example of a harlequin fetus. Note the parchment-like skin, the ectropion, and eclabium. The mouth with the eclabium sometimes has a fish-like appearance. The unyielding skin has resulted in cracking and fissuring at the corners of the mouth and the left hand is severely affected. This infant was treated with the oral administration of etretinate and topical use of Eucerin™. Following use of this approach there has been prolonged survival in a few infants.

1.229

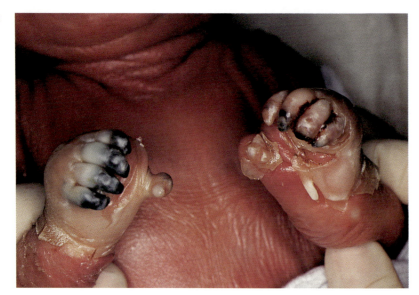

Figure 1.229. The hands of the same infant as in Figure 1.228. Note the pale, waxy, firm appearance and poorly developed digits which have become gangrenous. The nails may be hypoplastic or absent.

1.230

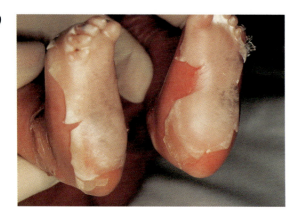

Figure 1.230. The feet of the same infant as in Figure 1.228 and 1.229 show the thick, rigid, hard, cracked skin and poorly developed toes with hypoplastic nails.

1.231

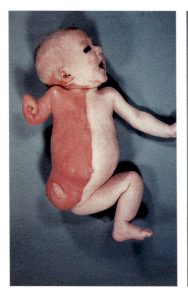
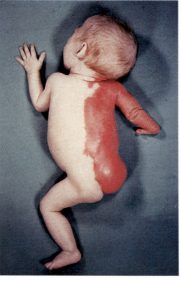

Figure 1.231. The CHILD syndrome is an X-linked dominant disorder (lethal to males) which is characterized by *congenital hemidysplasia*, with *ichthyosiform erythroderma*, and *limb defects*. The hallmark of the disorder is the sharp midline demarcation and the ipsilateral involvement of the skin and the extremities. The face is spared, and limb defects range in severity from hypoplasia of digits to complete agenesis of an extremity. In addition to the dermal and musculoskeletal involvement, other organs may be abnormal (viscera and occasionally the central nervous system).

1.232

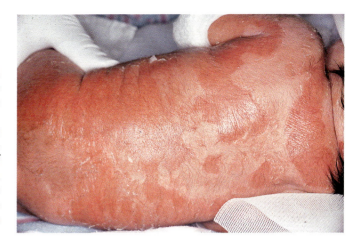

Figure 1.232. Following a spontaneous vaginal delivery in this term infant, desquamation of the skin was noted with the usual drying off in the delivery room. No bullae or blisters were noted. There was superficial desquamation over about 70% of the total body surface area. The Nikolsky's sign was positive. The diagnosis of "peeling skin syndrome" was confirmed by skin biopsy. This is an unusual congenital ichthyosis which is probably an autosomal recessive disease characterized by lifelong peeling of the epidermis with easy separation of the stratum corneum.

1.233

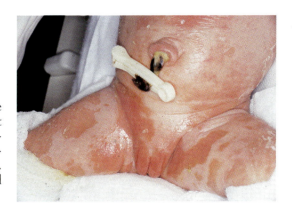

Figure 1.233. Another view of the same infant as in Figure 1.232 with the "peeling skin syndrome." This condition must be differentiated from non-bullous ichthyosiform erythroderma. Histopathologic features include intraepidermal separation between the stratum corneum and stratum granulosum. There may be a biochemical marker of moderate generalized aminoaciduria and low tryptophan levels.

OTHER DERMATOLOGIC PROBLEMS

1.234

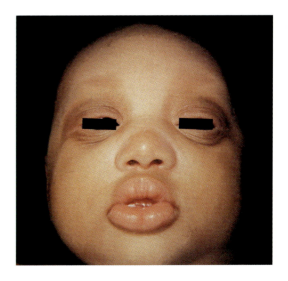

Figure 1.234. The typical facies of hypohidrotic (anhidrotic) ectodermal dysplasia is seen in this infant. Note the alopecia, absent eyebrows and eyelashes, square forehead with frontal bossing, hyperpigmented wrinkles around the eyes, flattened nasal bridge, and large conspicuous nostrils. There are wide cheek bones with depressed cheeks, thick everted lips, a prominent chin, and the ears may be small and pointed. These infants have a thin dry skin, decreased sweating, decreased tearing, and abnormal dentition. The nails are defective in a large percentage of these patients in that they may be thin, brittle, or ridged. If the absence of the sweat glands is generalized, they may have recurrent fever in high environmental temperatures.

1.235

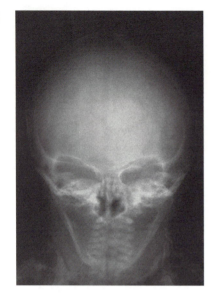

Figure 1.235. Radiograph of the face shows the typical hypoplasia of the maxillary alveolar processes and the lack of teeth (one of the hallmarks of hypohidrotic ectodermal dysplasia). Ectrodactyly-ectodermal dysplasia-clefting (EEC) syndrome should be considered in the differential diagnosis.

1.236

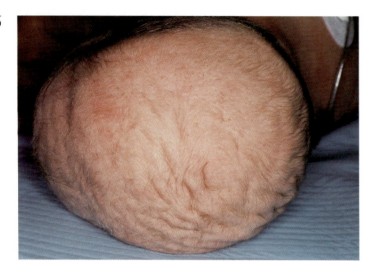

Figure 1.236. Cutis verticis gyrata is an unusual disorder characterized by coarse furrowing, most commonly of the vertex of the scalp and posterior aspect of the scalp and neck. The vertex usually has anteroposterior furrows whereas on the forehead and occiput they are transverse. The hair tends to be sparse on top of the folds and more profuse in the furrows. The entire scalp or only a small patch may have parallel folds of scalp skin furrowing with remarkable resemblance to the convolutions of the brain.

1.237

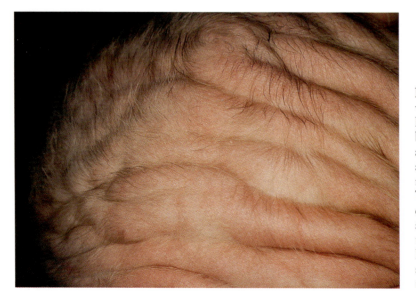

Figure 1.237. A close-up of cutis verticis gyrata in the same infant as in Figure 1.236. The condition is caused by an increase in dermal collagen and, as a result, excessive skin may buckle and form furrows and ridges that resemble gyri of the cerebral cortex. The condition may occur as a primary disorder without other associated abnormalities or it may be a manifestation of other pathology including Ehlers-Danlos syndrome, tuberous sclerosis, Apert's syndrome, hyperpituitarism, or pachydermomyositis.

1.238

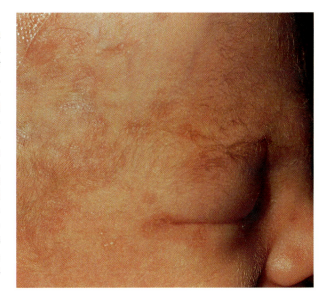

Figure 1.238. Neonatal lupus erythematosus is a unique variant of lupus erythematosus which occurs in infants born to mothers with or having a tendency for systemic lupus erythematosus, rheumatoid disease, etc. The majority of infants born to these mothers are usually normal, but they may have a lupus-like rash and lupus-associated hematologic and serologic abnormalities. The cutaneous lesions appear from birth (in two-thirds of cases) until about 12 weeks of age. The majority of infants have spontaneous resolution of the cutaneous lesions by about 6 to 12 months. In this infant note the diffuse erythema over the face and scalp, the scaly atrophic somewhat hypopigmented discoid lesions, and the alopecia which is a common finding in this disease. Cutaneous lesions of neonatal lupus erythematosus generally appear on the head and neck, extensor surfaces of the arms, and less frequently in other areas.

1.239

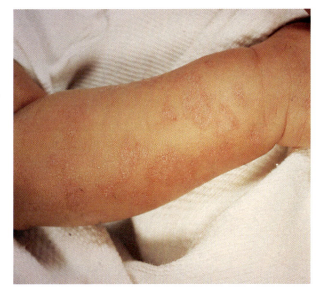

Figure 1.239. Sharply demarcated violaceous discoid lesions on the extensor surface of the forearm in another infant with neonatal lupus erythematosus. In neonatal lupus erythematosus about 15 to 30% of infants have congenital atrioventricular block, a complication which is usually irreversible with a high mortality rate (20 to 30% in the first few months of life.) During pregnancy the fetal ECG can be checked for heart block. Other systemic complications include cardiac malformations, hepatosplenomegaly, leukopenia, and thrombocytopenia. These infants have a positive Coombs' test and anti-Ro (SSA) antibodies are found in 95% of affected mother-infant pairs. Neonatal lupus was originally believed to be a transient disease but it is now apparent that continuing systemic involvement may occur.

1.240

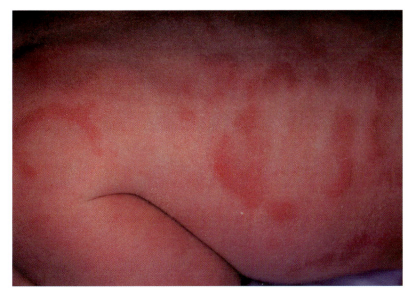

Figure 1.240. In erythema annulare centrifugum the lesions occur especially on the body, develop quickly, and can last for weeks. The lesions are erythematous and edematous, are of varying size and are partly ring-shaped in form. The centers of the lesions tend to fade and the lesions may spread out centrifugally and have a slightly scaly edge. The underlying etiology of this condition may be autoimmune disorders in the mother (such as lupus erythematosus), hypersensitivity to drugs, or fungal infection.

1.241

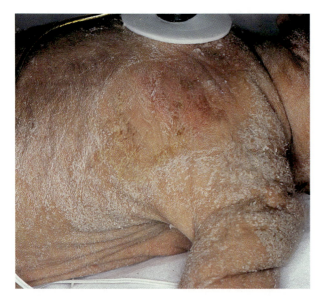

Figure 1.241. Exfoliative erythroderma occurred in this very small premature infant (birthweight 700 g) at 4 weeks of age following a blood transfusion for anemia at 3 weeks of age. He had a severe reaction and was critically ill for several days. There was marked blood eosinophilia and a diagnosis of graft-versus-host reaction was made. In acute graft-versus-host disease (GVHD) following transfusion, the findings include a generalized erythematous maculopapular exanthem with fine desquamation which later becomes a rough lamellar desquamation. There is no blister formation, and detachment of the nails may occur. Acute GVHD also affects the liver and may give abnormal liver function tests.

1.242

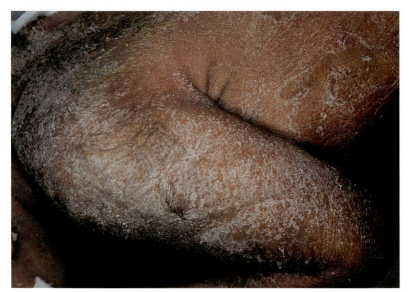

Figure 1.242. Close-up of the exfoliative erythroderma in the same infant as in Figure 1.241. This infant died at the age of 10 weeks, and at autopsy was found to have a primary immunodeficiency syndrome. Cutaneous manifestations of acute GVHD disease must be distinguished from drug eruptions or viral exanthems.

1.243

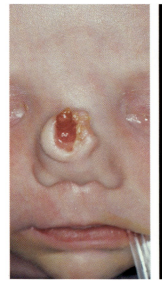 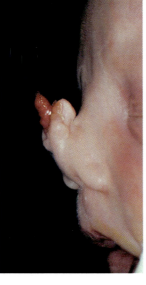

Figure 1.243. The diagnosis of a nasal dermoid in this infant was confirmed by biopsy. Dermoids are usually present at birth and occur particularly along the lines of embryonic fusion. They are most common on the head, especially around the eyes and the nose. Dermoid cysts may be attached to underlying structures. In any midline nasal mass, intracranial extension is common; thus, prior to removal of the mass, intracranial involvement should be excluded.

1.244

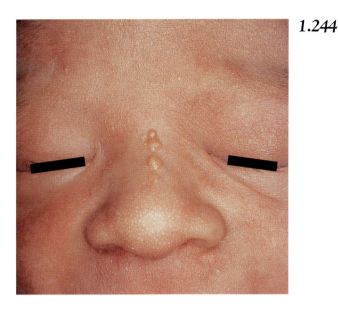

1.245

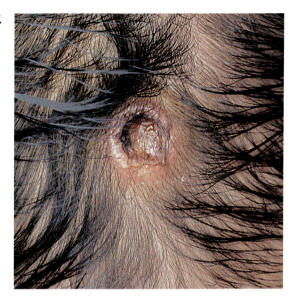

Figure 1.244. The diagnosis of a hamartoma of hair follicle origin was established by biopsy of the midline lesions of the nose in this infant.

Figure 1.245. Congenital self-healing reticulohistiocytosis (Hashimoto-Pritzker disease) is a rare disease usually present at birth or within the first few days of life. It is characterized by solitary or multiple reddish-brown, pink, or purplish papulovesicular lesions mainly on the scalp, face, trunk, and extremities. They tend to break down in the center, form ulcerated craters, and involute spontaneously within 2 to 3 months leaving white atrophic scars. Although the course is benign and self-limiting, it is important to differentiate this condition from histiocytosis X and other histiocytic conditions. Diagnosis is confirmed by skin biopsy.

Figure 1.246. In juvenile xanthogranulomatosis the lesions are present at birth. They are characterized by solitary or multiple yellow to reddish-brown papules and nodules of the face, scalp, neck, and sometimes the sublingual areas and the proximal portions of the extremities or trunk. The lesions may enlarge and become bright yellow as they mature. Spontaneous regression usually occurs in the first year of life. Diagnosis is confirmed by biopsy which shows histiocytes of the non-Langerhans' cells and the presence of Touton giant cells. The lesions are harmless but should not be overlooked since there is an apparent association with neurofibromatosis. (Kenny, J.)

1.246

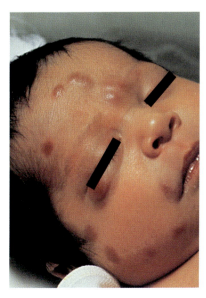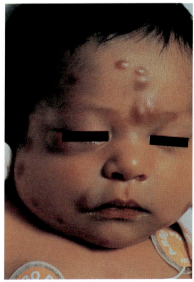

1.247

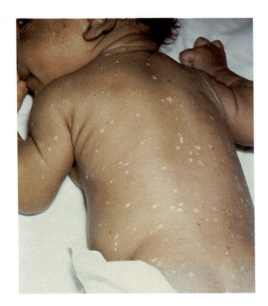

Figure 1.247. Skin lesions, present at birth in this infant with histiocytosis X, on biopsy showed the typical finding of the presence of histiocytes of the Langerhans' cell type and eosinophilia. The term "congenital histiocytosis" includes Letterer-Siwe disease, Hand-Schüller-Christian disease, and eosinophilic granuloma. These conditions are now grouped together as histiocytosis X.

1.248

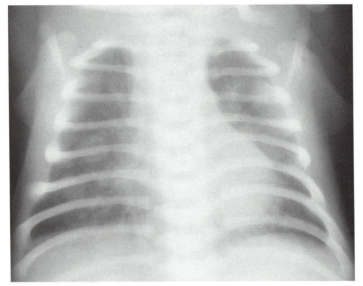

Figure 1.248. Chest radiograph in an infant at the age of 3 days with histiocytosis. Note the infiltrative coin-like lesions which are typical with pulmonary involvement in histiocytosis X. The presence of pulmonary and other systemic involvement worsens the prognosis.

1.249

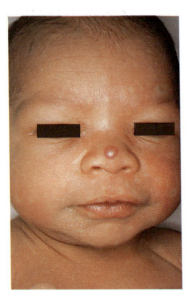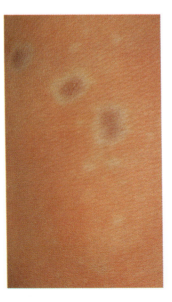

Figure 1.249. In this infant with congenital generalized fibromatosis, on the left note the lesion on the nose and the purplish area surrounded by a pale halo above the left eyebrow. On the right is a close-up of the lesions on the back of the same infant. The infants may also have firm hard nodules in the skin and subcutaneous tissue. In congenital generalized fibromatosis it is necessary to check the long bones and lungs for systemic involvement.

1.250

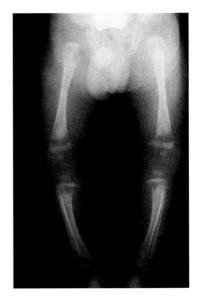

Figure 1.250. Radiograph of the long bones in another infant with congenital generalized fibromatosis showing the areas of erosion due to the presence of generalized fibromata.

1.251

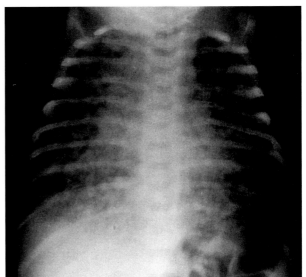

Figure 1.251. Chest radiograph showing extensive pulmonary involvement in an infant with congenital generalized fibromatosis. The presence of pulmonary involvement signifies a poor prognosis.

Chapter 2
Perinatal Infection

The immediate and long-term effects of perinatal infection are a major problem throughout the world. Perinatal infection is relatively common among the over 4 million births per year in the United States but the incidence is dependent upon the organism. One percent of newborn infants excrete cytomegalovirus. Fifteen percent are infected with *Chlamydia trachomatis*; one-third develop conjunctivitis and one-sixth, pneumonia. One to eight per 1,000 live births develop bacterial sepsis. In utero or perinatal infection with herpes simplex virus, *Toxoplasma gondii* and varicella-zoster virus occurs in about 1 per 1,000 live births and the sequelae may be severe. In-utero acquired infection may result in resorption of the embryo, abortion, stillbirth, malformation, intrauterine growth retardation, prematurity, and the numerous untoward sequelae associated with chronic infection. Infection acquired at or soon after birth may lead to death or persistent postnatal infection. Some infections may be inapparent at birth and present years later with signs (e.g., choreoretinitis of *T. gondii*, hearing loss of rubella virus, and immunologic defects of HIV). Early diagnosis and aggressive treatment of infection during pregnancy may lower the associated morbidity and mortality rates substantially.

2.1 BACTERIAL INFECTION

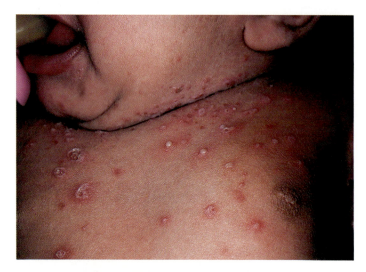

Figure 2.1. Staphylococcal furunculosis developed in this infant at the age of 6 days. A Gram stain of the material in the lesions showed numerous polymorphonuclear leukocytes and gram-positive cocci. The culture grew *Staphylococcus aureus*. Included in the differential diagnosis of these lesions are transient neonatal pustular melanosis and herpes.

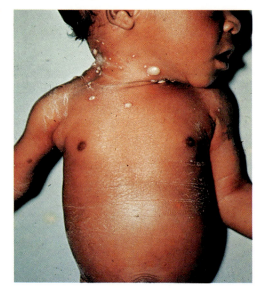

Figure 2.2. Staphylococcal pyoderma of the neck in an infant at the age of 8 days.

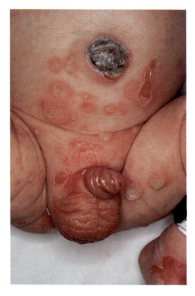

Figure 2.3. Bullous impetigo (pemphigus neonatorum) in a newborn infant at the age of 6 days. This infection may occur as early as the second day or as late as two weeks of life and may demonstrate both bullous and impetiginous lesions. It is most commonly due to a staphylococcal infection but, on occasion, is caused by *Streptococcus*. The lesions are more common in moist, warm areas such as the axillary folds of the neck or the groin and present as superficial bullae which are wrinkled, become flaccid, and rupture easily producing ulcers which become crusted. Note the impetigo of the umbilical area.

2.4

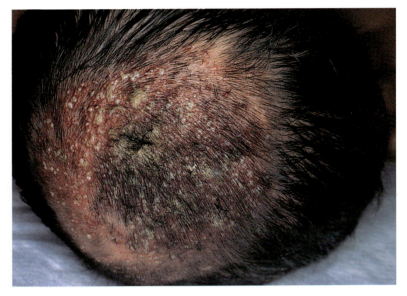

Figure 2.4. Scalp abscesses developed at 12 hours of age. Note the distribution over the area of the caput. In such an infant the diagnoses of herpes simplex and *Staphylococcus aureus* infection should be considered. Cultures from the lesions and the blood in this infant were positive for *Staphylococcus aureus*. The mother developed fever 24 hours postpartum, and *Staphylococcus aureus* was cultured from the episiotomy.

2.5

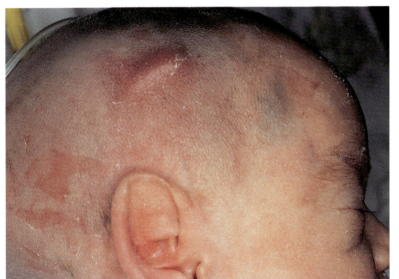

Figure 2.5. This nosocomial scalp abscess developed in a premature infant (birthweight 1000 g) at the age of 12 days. *Staphylococcus aureus* was cultured from both the abscess and the blood. The parietal area is the most frequent site for scalp abscess. Scalp abscesses frequently occur with the use of repeated scalp vein infusions.

2.6

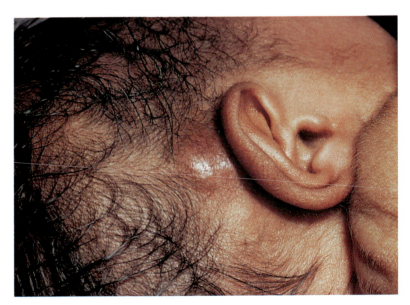

Figure 2.6. Postauricular scalp abscess in an infant due to *Staphylococcus aureus* infection as a result of forceps application.

2.7

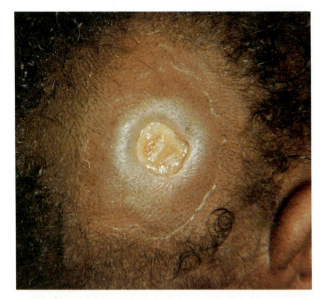

Figure 2.7. Healing staphylococcal abscess resulting from application of forceps during delivery. These usually are noted over the parietal area. Skin abrasions caused by application of forceps or scalp electrodes for fetal monitoring may become secondarily infected, resulting in the development of a scalp abscess.

2.8

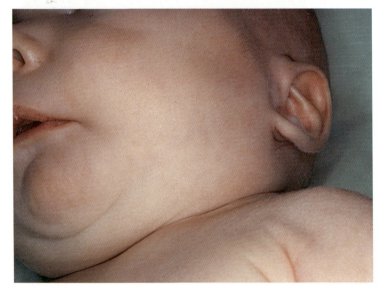

Figure 2.8. Staphylococcal parotitis in a two week old infant. Note the swelling over the parotid area.

2.9

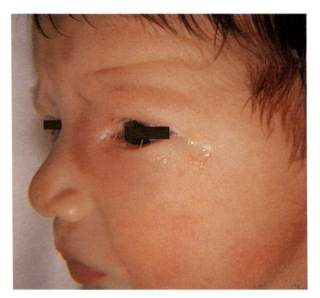

Figure 2.9. Acute staphylococcal dacryocystitis developed in this neonate at the age of 2 weeks. Note that in addition to the swelling over the lacrimal gland, there is conjunctival inflammatory change. Staphylococcal infection is the most common cause of this infection, but it may occur with infection by *Streptococcus* or *Neisseria*.

2.10

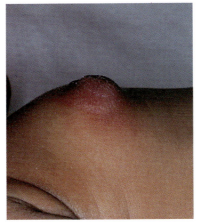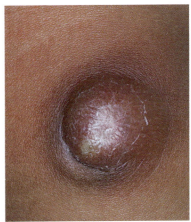

Figure 2.10. Breast abscess in a neonate due to *Staphylococcus aureus*. In the left figure note the infection as seen in the lateral view. A close-up of the abscess is shown in the right figure.

2.11

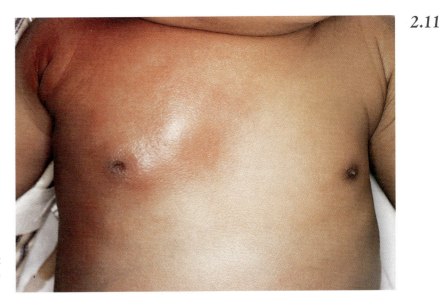

Figure 2.11. Mastitis of the right breast with abscess formation and cellulitis of the chest.

2.12

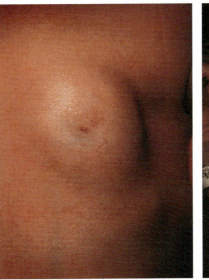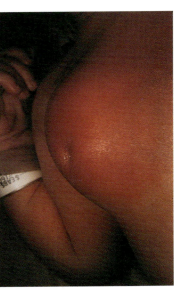

Figure 2.12. On the left note the normal physiologic engorgement of the breast. On the right there is a mastitis secondary to *Escherichia coli* infection. Although the most common cause of mastitis in the neonate is staphylococcal infection, other organisms may be responsible.

2.13

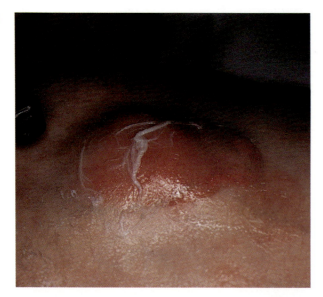

Figure 2.13. This large abscess over the xiphoid area developed at the age of 10 days in a neonate who had methicillin-sensitive *Staphylococcus aureus* sepsis.

2.14

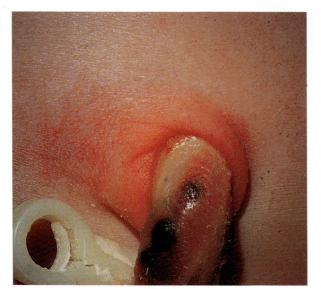

Figure 2.14. Staphylococcal omphalitis and funisitis in a neonate. The erythema of the skin surrounding the umbilical cord is due to omphalitis. Funisitis represents infection of the umbilical cord per se. Note the redness of the umbilical cord.

2.15

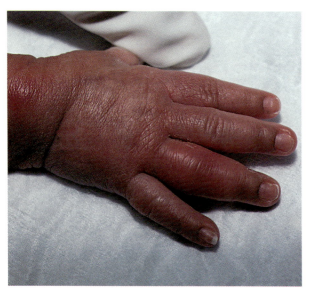

Figure 2.15. Nosocomial infection causing an abscess of the right wrist and cellulitis of the 4th finger in a premature infant (birth weight 1100 g) at the age of 35 days. This infant had methicillin-resistant *Staphylococcus aureus* bacteremia. There was no osseous involvement. The infant was successfully treated with vancomycin.

Figure 2.16. Acute osteomyelitis of the distal end of the right femur presenting with marked swelling of the right knee joint. Blood culture was positive for *Staphylococcus aureus*. The diagnosis of osteomyelitis must be excluded in any neonate with a swollen joint or who is reluctant to move a limb spontaneously. Neonatal osteomyelitis may occur 1) by direct inoculation, 2) by extension from infection in surrounding soft tissues (e.g., infected cephalhematoma), 3) by transplacental extension from maternal bacteremia (e.g., congenital syphilis), and 4) by blood-borne dissemination in neonatal septicemia (the major cause of neonatal osteomyelitis by metastatic seeding of the skeletal system through the nutrient arteries).

2.16

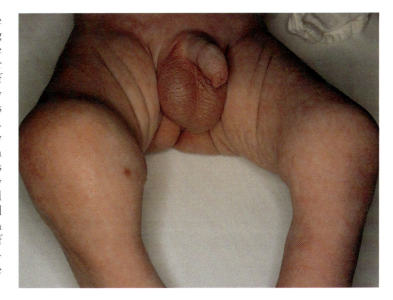

2.17

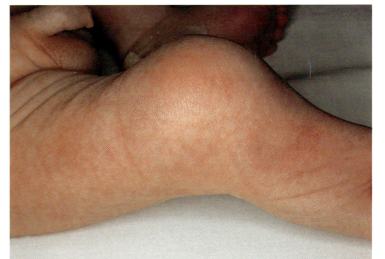

Figure 2.17. Lateral view of the right knee joint in the same infant demonstrates the marked joint swelling. The hips or knees or both are involved in 70% of cases of neonatal osteomyelitis. The higher incidence of sepsis in premature infants may contribute to the much higher incidence of osteomyelitis in premature infants.

Figure 2.18. Radiographs of the same infant showing, left to right, *A)* marked swelling of the soft tissues and the joint with little evidence of bony change, *B)* two days later note early changes at the distal end of the femur, and *C)* marked improvement after 1 month of treatment. Unlike older children in which radiologic changes are delayed for several weeks, in the neonate changes of bone destruction are almost always present by the 7th to 10th day of illness. Capsular distention or widening of the joint is common. The reparative phase begins within 2 weeks after onset of infection, and the entire process from the first signs of rarefaction to restoration of the cortical structures may last no longer than 2 months.

2.18

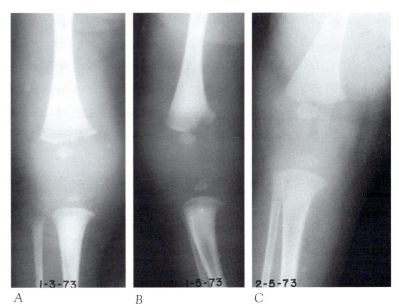

A   B   C

2.19

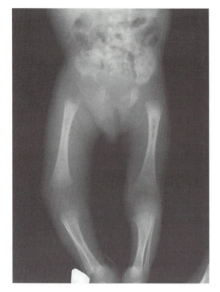

Figure 2.19. Osteomyelitis of the proximal end of the right femur with marked bony changes. Note the marked increase in the size of the hip joint. This again demonstrates that joint swelling may be the first indication of the development of osteomyelitis. The reason for the common involvement of joints in the neonatal period is that sinusoidal vessels, termed transphyseal vessels, connect the two separate circulatory systems seen in the bones of older children (the metaphyseal loops which derive from the diaphyseal nutrient artery and the epiphyseal vessels which course through the epiphyseal cartilage canals). With skeletal maturation the transphyseal vessels obliterate (8 to 18 months) and the epiphyseal and metaphyseal systems become totally separate.

2.20

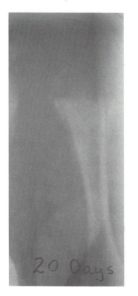 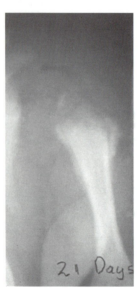 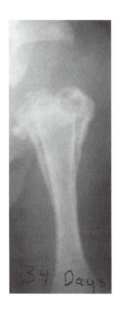

Figure 2.20. Neonatal osteomyelitis due to *Proteus mirabilis* infection. Although *Staphylococcus aureus* is the most common etiologic agent of osteomyelitis in the neonate, many other organisms such as group B *Streptococcus, E. coli, Klebsiella, Salmonella* and *Candida* have been implicated.

2.21

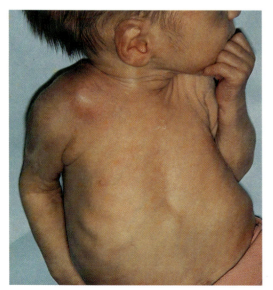

Figure 2.21. Osteomyelitis usually occurs in the long bones, but in the neonate frequently occurs in other bones such as the clavicle and ribs. This infant demonstrates inflammation and swelling over the right clavicle due to a staphylococcal osteomyelitis.

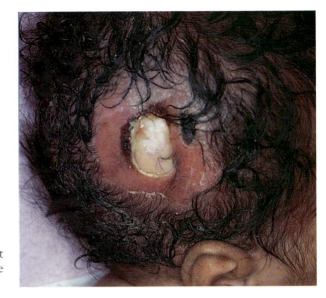

2.22

Figure 2.22. Severe scalp defect occurring as a result of an underlying staphylococcal osteomyelitis of the skull.

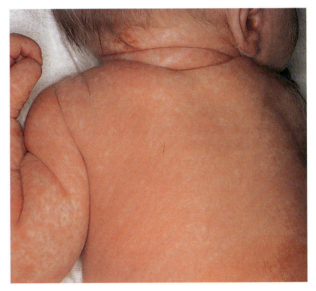

2.23

Figure 2.23. This infant presented with fever, lethargy and poor feeding at 4 days of age. He then developed a generalized rash which resembled scarlatina. Blood culture was positive for a *Staphylococcus aureus* phage type which produces an erythrogenic toxin, hence the appearance of the rash.

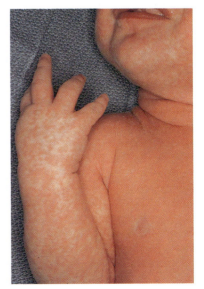

2.24

Figure 2.24. Close-up of the rash in the same infant.

2.25

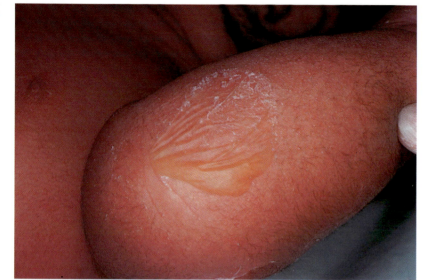

Figure 2.25. This infant who developed a mild scalded skin syndrome (toxic epidermal necrolysis; Ritter's disease) at the age of seven days had *Staphylococcus aureus* sepsis (methicillin-sensitive). Note the large bullae at this very early stage of the staphylococcal scalded skin syndrome. This is rapidly progressive. The skin is erythematous with vesicular and bullous formation, and there is widespread wrinkling and loosening of the epidermis, which results in the scalded skin appearance.

2.26

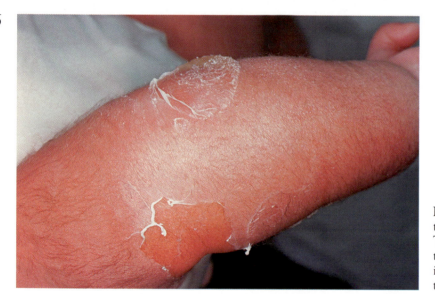

Figure 2.26. In the same infant there is rupture of the bullae. These infants present with the typical Nikolsky's sign in that there is skin exfoliation which peels on touch.

2.27

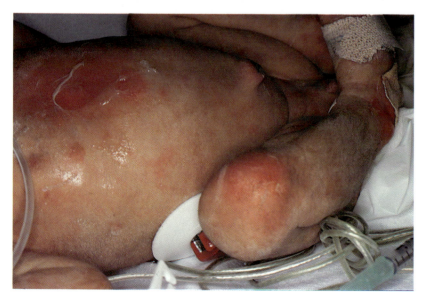

Figure 2.27. In this infant with the staphylococcal scalded skin syndrome, the bullous lesions have ruptured, resulting in the scalded skin appearance. Staphylococcal scalded skin syndrome is also known as Ritter's disease.

2.28

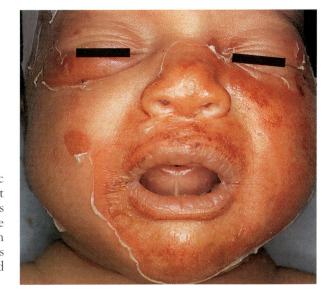

Figure 2.28. This infant had rapid progressive toxic epidermal necrolysis. The face is usually affected first and progression may rapidly become generalized. This condition is most commonly due to phage group type II staphylococci, and the toxin from the organism causes the severe exfoliative dermatitis which results in the systemic manifestations of fever, instability and water loss.

2.29

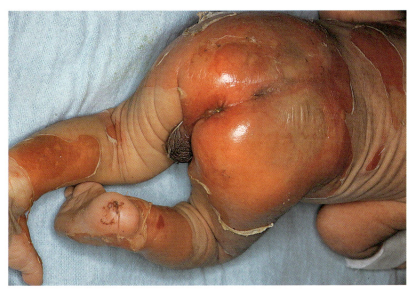

Figure 2.29. The body, buttocks and lower extremities of the same infant showing the very extensive "scalding" of the skin.

2.30

Figure 2.30. This infant has necrotizing fasciitis of the abdominal wall, which is a rapidly progressive acute necrotizing infection of the skin, subcutaneous tissue, muscle, and fascia. Necrotizing fasciitis usually presents as an area of cellulitis with fever, redness, and edema. It rapidly progresses to central patches of bluish discoloration followed by ulceration, gangrene, and toxicity. Necrotizing fasciitis is a surgical emergency as it is rapidly fatal if not treated aggressively by widespread incision and debridement. Infection in this condition has been associated with *Staphylococcus aureus*, anaerobic *Streptococcus*, *Bacteroides* and *Proteus*.

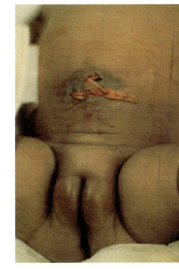
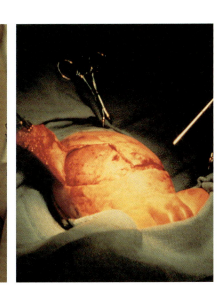

2.31

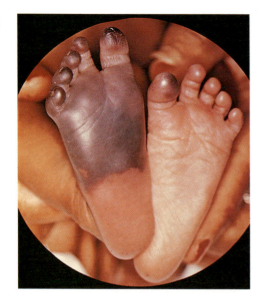

Figure 2.31. Staphylococcal sepsis resulting in gangrene of the right foot and left big toe. Umbilical catheters were not used in this infant.

2.32

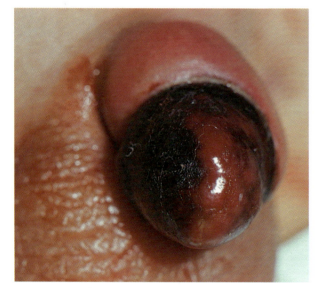

Figure 2.32. Forty-eight hours after circumcision at the age of 3 days, this infant developed cellulitis and inflammatory change of the glans and penis. There was thrombocytopenia and positive blood culture for *Staphylococcus aureus*.

2.33

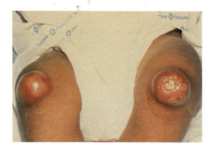

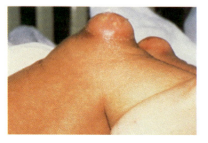

Figure 2.33. Bilateral prepatellar bursitis in a very active neonate who abraded her knees. Aspiration of the purulent material yielded group B *Streptococcus*. The knee joints, per se, were not affected. This complication is extremely rare. (Edwards, M.)

2.34

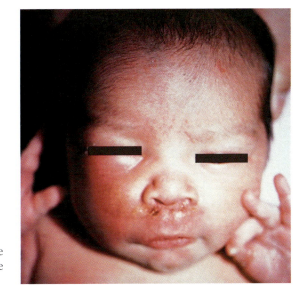

Figure 2.34. Marked cellulitis of the right side of the face in a neonate with group B streptococcal infection. There was a positive blood culture for group B *Streptococcus*.

2.35

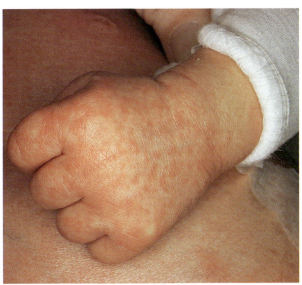

Figure 2.35. Beta hemolytic streptococcal sepsis is rare in neonates. This infant had a generalized scarlatiniform rash. Cultures were positive for group A *Streptococcus* (bacitracin-sensitive).

2.36

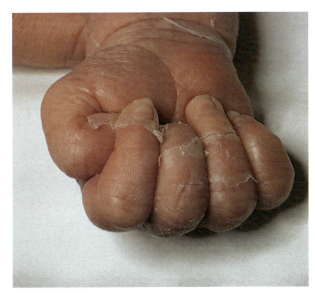

Figure 2.36. In the same infant as in Figure 2.35, note the marked desquamation of the skin 1 week later. This is similar to the typical desquamation in scarlatina in older children.

2.37

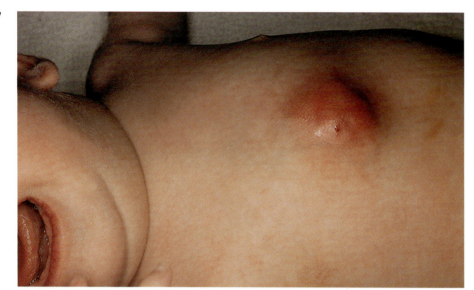

Figure 2.37. This infant with streptococcal sepsis developed cellulitis over a prominent xiphoid process.

2.38

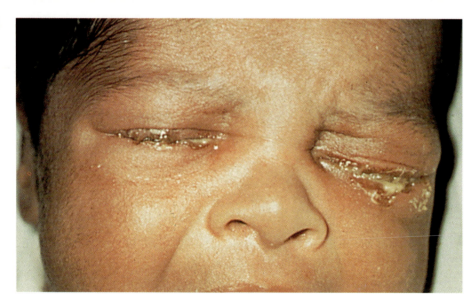

Figure 2.38. Gonococcal ophthalmia neonatorum in an infant at the age of 4 days. With prophylaxis this disease is rarely seen today. The most common cause of neonatal ophthalmia at the present time is staphylococcal infection.

2.39

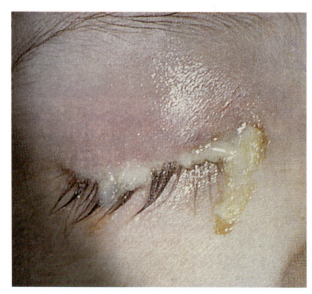

Figure 2.39. Close-up of an infant with marked purulent discharge caused by gonococcal ophthalmia neonatorum. Even with Credé's method, occasionally a breakthrough of gonococcal infection does occur in infants in that they may develop a mild conjunctivitis at the age of 7 to 14 days which is positive for *Neisseria.*

2.40

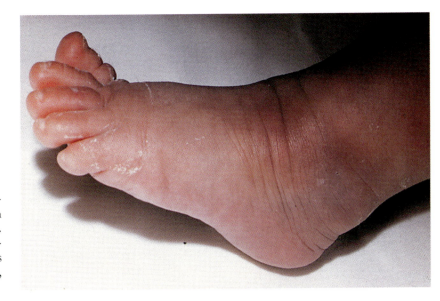

Figure 2.40. Gonococcal arthritis of the left ankle joint in an infant at the age of 2 weeks. As in the adult, neonatal gonococcal infection generally affects the large joints (knee, ankle, etc.).

2.41

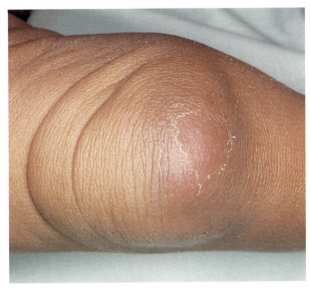

Figure 2.41. *Haemophilus influenzae* cellulitis of the prepatellar area in a neonate. Note the violaceous discoloration. This is very typical of *Haemophilus influenzae* cellulitis. The infant may be very ill with this type of infection. Cellulitis can occur as a result of infection with many other organisms.

2.42

Figure 2.42. In this infant with congenital listeriosis, skin lesions were present over the entire body at birth. These increased in number. The infant had severe respiratory distress and had a congenital pneumonia due to listeriosis. The amniotic fluid was brown in color and *Listeria monocytogenes* was cultured from both skin lesions and the blood. Chocolate-brown amniotic fluid is typically seen in listeriosis. If meconium staining is reported in premature infants of less than 32 weeks gestation listerial infection may be the cause. A good site for culture of the organism is the meconium or stool.

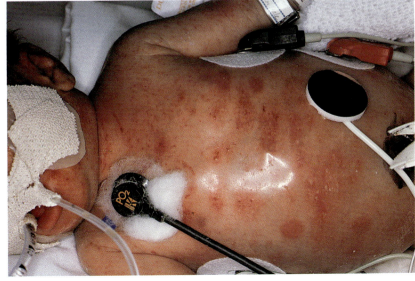

2.43

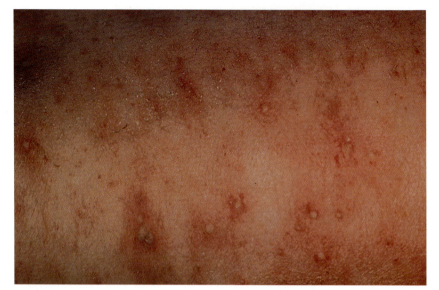

Figure 2.43. Close-up of the skin lesions of the same infant as in Figure 2.42. Note the macules, papules and vesicles. In the septicemic form of listeriosis, a cutaneous eruption of miliary abscesses resembling papules, pustules, or papulo-pustules may occur over the entire body with a predilection for the back. Culture of the lesions, the blood, or cerebrospinal fluid usually reveals *Listeria monocytogenes* as the offending agent.

2.44

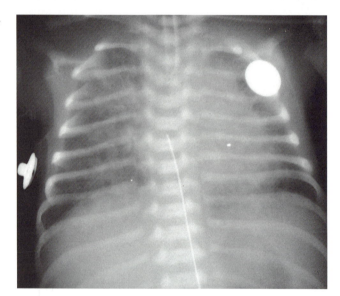

Figure 2.44. Chest radiograph in an infant who presented with severe respiratory distress from congenital pneumonia due to congenital listeriosis. The radiograph is not specific in that there may be peribronchial to wide-spread infiltration. In long-standing cases a coarse mottled or nodular pattern may be present.

2.45

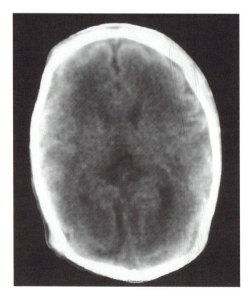

Figure 2.45. CT scan of a neonate who had listerial meningitis. Note the loss of morphology due to loss of white and gray matter differentiation. The villi are flattened out and there is evidence of some atrophy with fluid in the subarachnoid spaces. Listerial meningitis may present with early-onset disease (up to 7 days of age) usually associated with serotype I or late-onset disease (mean age 12 to 14 days) usually associated with serotype IV. Prognosis is poor in early-onset disease as seen in this infant. Note that late-onset listerial infection presents with fever in 90 to 95% of cases whereas hypothermia is much more common in other neonatal infections.

2.46

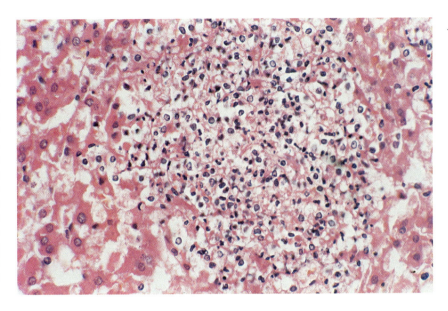

Figure 2.46. Histologic section of the liver shows the typical necrotic lesion of granuloma infantisepticum. Human listeriosis is characterized by the formation of miliary granulomas and focal necrosis or suppuration in the affected tissues. *Listeria* organisms are detectable in the necrotic foci. These lesions of granuloma infantisepticum are classically observed in generalized listeriosis. Massive involvement of the liver is predominant, but the lesions are also seen in the spleen, adrenal glands, lungs and throughout other tissues.

2.47

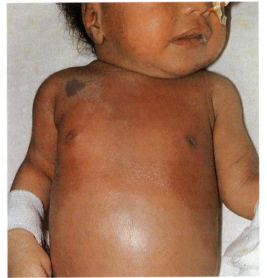

Figure 2.47. This term infant developed cellulitis of the upper chest and back at the age of 9 days. Note the very definite line of demarcation in the chest. At the same time the infant developed a purplish area over the infraclavicular and scapular areas. A sepsis evaluation was performed and cultures were positive for a gram-negative infection due to *Paracolobactrum*. (*Paracolobactrum* is in the same group as *Escherichia*, differing in that it has delayed fermentation of lactose. At the present time, it is included in the *Salmonella-Arizona* group of Enterobacteriaceae.) Prior to the report of the blood culture, differential diagnosis included erysipelas, as the line of demarcation was slightly raised, and gram-negative sepsis due to *Achromobacter*.

2.48

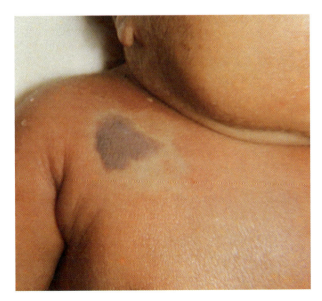

Figure 2.48. A close-up of the lesion 1 day later in the same infant as in Figure 2.47. The lesion is more violaceous in color and the diagnosis of fasciitis was made.

2.49

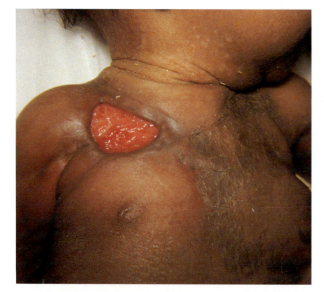

Figure 2.49. In the same infant as in Figure 2.47 and 2.48, the infraclavicular lesion broke down with severe damage to the underlying subcutaneous tissue and muscle ulceration developed; this healed with scarring over time. Note the lesion at the age of 37 days.

2.50

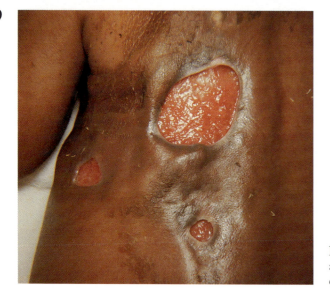

Figure 2.50. The same infant as in Figure 2.47 to 2.49 at the age of 57 days showing the lesions with breakdown and healing on the back.

2.51

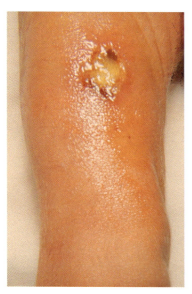 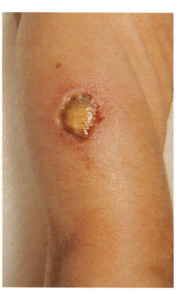

Figure 2.51. Typical "fried egg" appearance (necrotic center with surrounding inflammation) of skin lesions associated with *Pseudomonas* infection are seen in this 4-day-old neonate. This lesion developed at the site of a Vitamin K injection. *Pseudomonas aeruginosa* is usually a cause of late-onset disease in infants who are presumably infected via equipment, aqueous solutions or, on occasion, the hands of health care personnel.

The same infant with *Pseudomonas* infection shows healing at the age of nine days. Note the necrotic center. These lesions are indolent and slow healing.

Figure 2.52. This infant with *Pseudomonas aeruginosa* sepsis and meningitis was acutely ill and had convulsions. He developed multiple skin lesions at the age of 12 days. Convulsions were controlled with difficulty and the infant died one week later. Although it is very uncommon, *Pseudomonas* conjunctivitis (a very purulent conjunctivitis) may be a devastating disease and if not promptly recognized and treated there may be rapid progression to septicemia, shock, and death. *Pseudomonas* sepsis may also cause purpura fulminans (thrombocytopenia, and clinical and laboratory signs of disseminated intravascular coagulopathy).

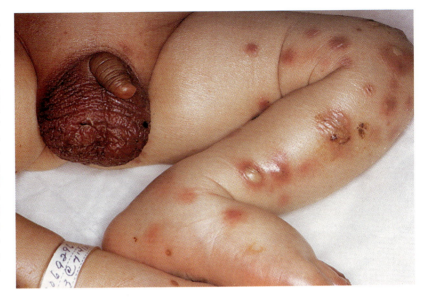

2.52

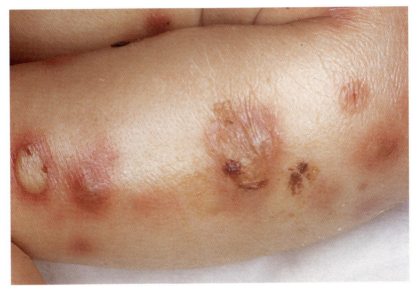

2.53

Figure 2.53. Close-up view of the typical lesions in the same infant. The cutaneous eruption in *Pseudomonas* infection consists of pearly vesicles on an erythematous background, which rapidly become purulent green or hemorrhagic. When the lesion ruptures, a circumscribed ulcer with a necrotic base appears and may persist surrounded by a purplish cellulitis.

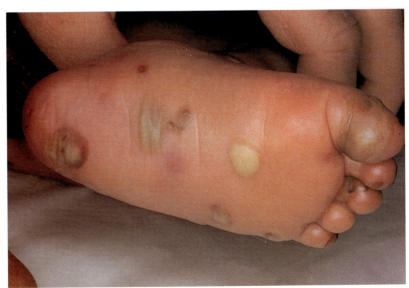

2.54

Figure 2.54. The typical lesions were also present on the soles of the feet. These lesions should not be confused with the lesions of syphilitic pemphigus.

2.55

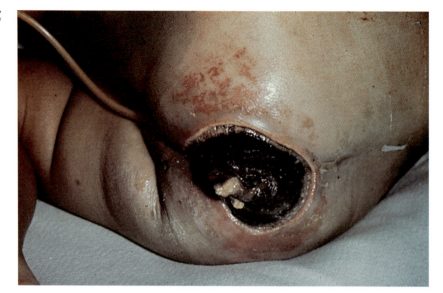

Figure 2.55. These gangrenous lesions associated with bacteremia caused by *Pseudomonas aeruginosa* demonstrate how devastating this infection can be.

2.56

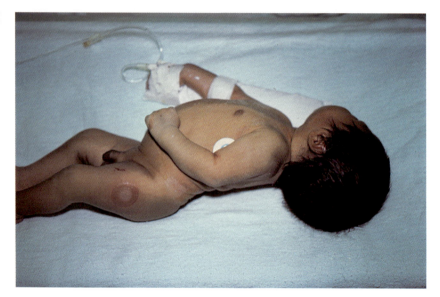

Figure 2.56. The typical opisthotonic appearance in an infant with neonatal tetanus. Note the head retraction, arching of the spine, and the hyperextension of the extremities resulting in a rigid posture. Neonatal tetanus is caused by gram-positive anaerobic spores of *Clostridium tetani*, present in the soil and in animal and human feces. Infection usually occurs after contamination of the umbilical stump that may result from unsanitary delivery or unclean handling of the cord. In developing countries the incidence of neonatal tetanus remains high.

2.57

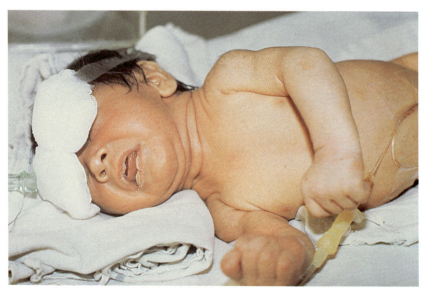

Figure 2.57. This infant with neonatal tetanus has the typical trismus giving rise to the risus sardonicus and tetanic spasm. Especially note the hands. Risus sardonicus is a grinning expression produced by spasm of the facial muscles.

2.58

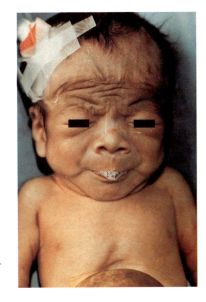

Figure 2.58. This infant with an omphalocele was delivered by a lay midwife under poor hygienic conditions. He developed tetanus at the age of 4 days and shows the typical risus sardonicus. (Cabrera-Meza, G.)

2.59

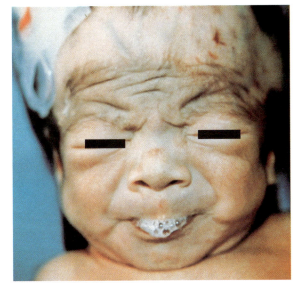

Figure 2.59. Close-up view of the face of the same infant as in Figure 2.58 showing the risus sardonicus. Note the excess secretions. (Cabrera-Meza, G.)

2.60

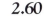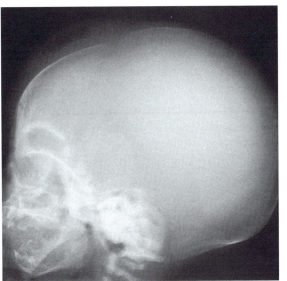

Figure 2.60. Lateral radiograph of a skull. Note the gas in a scalp abscess caused by a localized infection by a gas-forming organism.

2.61

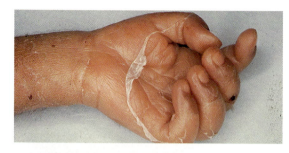

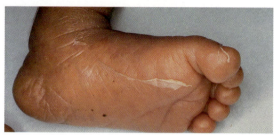

Figure 2.61. Note the desquamation of the palms and soles in a neonate. There were no other dermatologic lesions elsewhere. The VDRL (Venereal Disease Research Laboratory) test showed maternal blood to be reactive with a titer of 1:32 and the infant had a titer of 1:1024. Lesions on the palms and soles should be considered syphilitic until proven otherwise. The spectrum of cutaneous lesions which occur in 30 to 40% of infants with congenital syphilis can be extremely variable. There may be mild desquamation, annular or circinate lesions or vesiculobullous manifestations.

2.62

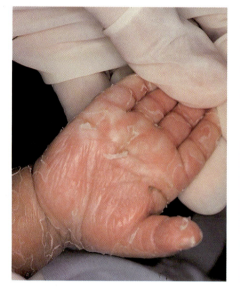

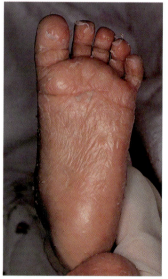

Figure 2.62. Desquamation on the palms and soles with no rash or desquamation elsewhere is very suggestive of congenital syphilis. The palms and soles may be fissured and erythematous and, as a result of subcutaneous edema, may have a shiny appearance.

2.63

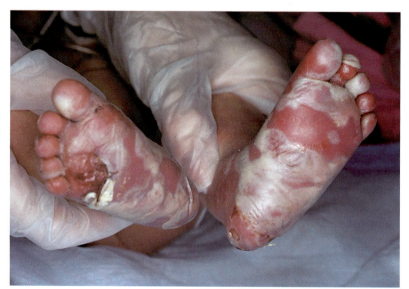

Figure 2.63. Syphilitic pemphigus showing the large vesiculobullous hemorrhagic lesions on the soles of both feet. These lesions are relatively rare but, especially when seen on the palms and soles, are highly diagnostic of this disease. The lesions may contain a cloudy hemorrhagic fluid that teems with organisms and is highly contagious. With bullous lesions such as these, other dermatologic diagnoses should be excluded (bullous impetigo, epidermolysis bullosa, congenital bullous ichthyosiform erythroderma, etc.).

2.64

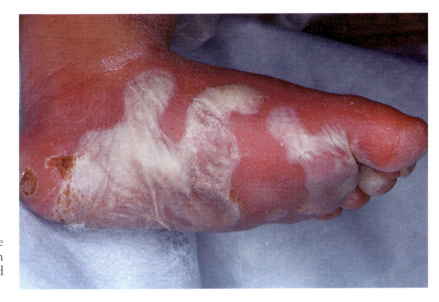

Figure 2.64. A close-up of the foot of the same infant as in Figure 2.63 shows both bullae and ulcerated areas on the sole.

2.65

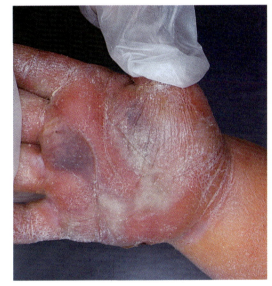

Figure 2.65. The same infant as in Figure 2.63 had bullae and ulcerations on the palms of both hands. When bullae rupture, they leave a denuded area that can undergo extensive maceration and crusting. It is unusual to see the bullae at birth as the majority have ruptured in utero.

2.66

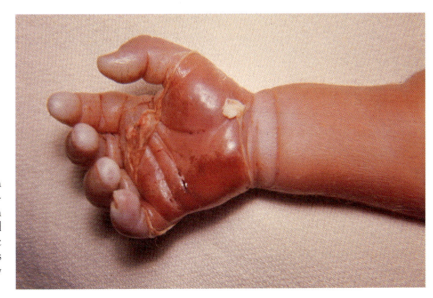

Figure 2.66. This infant with congenital syphilis had vesiculobullous hemorrhagic lesions which ruptured in utero and presented with the typical raw, hemorrhagic appearance of the palms and soles at birth. These lesions are highly infectious.

2.67

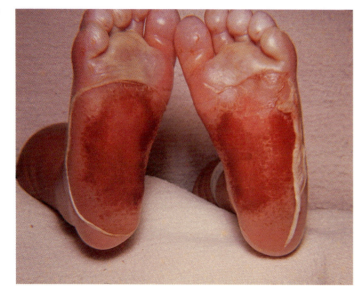

Figure 2.67. The raw hemorrhagic appearance of the lesions on the soles of the same infant as in Figure 2.66. In general, the more florid the manifestations of congenital syphilis at birth, the worse the prognosis.

2.68

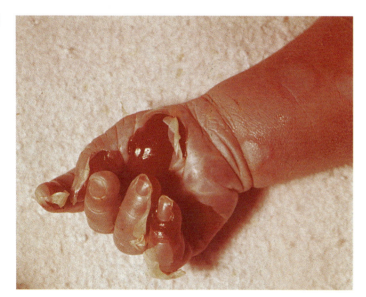

Figure 2.68. Characteristic circinate lesions involving the distal forearm in congenital syphilis. Syphilitic pemphigus of the palm is also present. The cutaneous manifestations may appear as large round or oval maculopapular (circinate) lesions. These are comparable to the lesions seen in secondary syphilis in the adult. It is unusual for them to be present at birth as they usually present between the age of 3 to 6 weeks in infants with congenital syphilis.

2.69

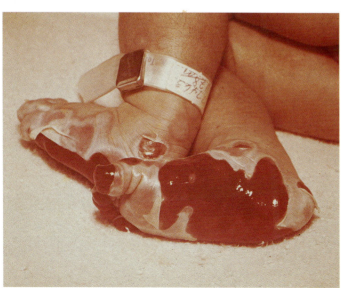

Figure 2.69. Circinate lesions and syphilitic pemphigus of the soles present at birth in the same infant as in Figure 2.68.

2.70

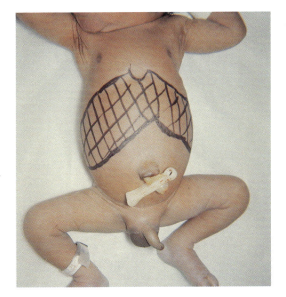

Figure 2.70. Marked hepatosplenomegaly in an infant with congenital syphilis. Hepatomegaly occurs in 50 to 60% of affected infants. It is frequently associated with jaundice, anemia, splenomegaly and ascites. In the spectrum of congenital syphilis there may be no clinical signs of disease at birth or there may be many clinical manifestations which include intrauterine growth retardation, skin manifestations, hepatosplenomegaly, jaundice, anemia, thrombocytopenia, and osseous changes.

2.71

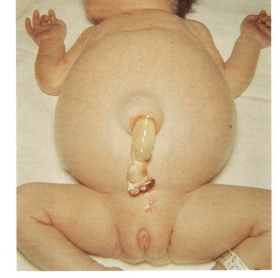

Figure 2.71. This infant with massive ascites secondary to congenital syphilis associated with respiratory distress, improved dramatically after abdominal paracentesis. This degree of ascites caused dystocia, necessitating a cesarean delivery.

2.72

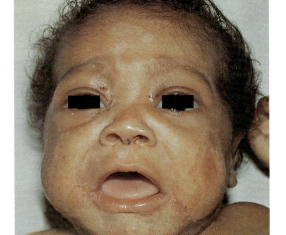

Figure 2.72. In an infant aged 6 weeks with the typical findings of congenital syphilis, note the circinate lesions over the forehead, the excoriation at the nose due to rhinitis, and the cheilitis at the corners of the mouth. Rhinitis ("snuffles") usually appears between the 2nd to 6th week of life and is the result of ulceration of the nasal mucosa. When the ulceration is deep enough to involve the cartilage of the nasal bone, the architecture is destroyed, thus giving rise to the classic saddle nose deformity. Mucous membrane patches are seen in approximately one-third of infants with congenital syphilis. At the mucocutaneous junctions these lesions tend to weep and may cause fissures (cheilitis) which often extend from the lips in a radiating fashion over the surrounding skin. When deep, these lesions may leave residual scars (rhagades).

2.73

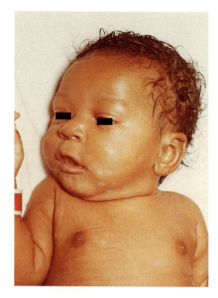

Figure 2.73. This infant developed a skin rash of congenital syphilis at the age of 7 weeks. These annular and circinate lesions healed but left areas of hypopigmentation. This type of cutaneous lesion, rarely present at birth, generally develops as a dark pink or red rash from the age of 3 to 6 weeks; it gradually fades to a coppery-brown lesion which disappears over a period of 1 to 2 months but often leaves an area of hyperpigmentation or hypopigmentation. The lesions may occur on any part of the body, but are usually most pronounced on the face and the dorsal surface of the trunk and legs.

2.74

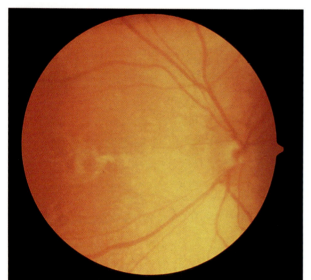

Figure 2.74. Congenital syphilitic chorioretinitis of the right eye. Note the abnormal scarring in the macular area. Optic atrophy, if present, is usually seen in conjunction with neurosyphilis. These findings are extremely rare in congenital syphilis. Other stigmata of congenital syphilis present much later. The deciduous teeth of children with early congenital syphilis are prone to caries but show no other abnormality. The stigmata of Hutchinson's triad (Hutchinson's incisors, interstitial keratitis, and eighth nerve deafness) occur later. Dental changes of Hutchinson's incisors and Moon's (mulberry) molars occur with secondary dentition.

2.75

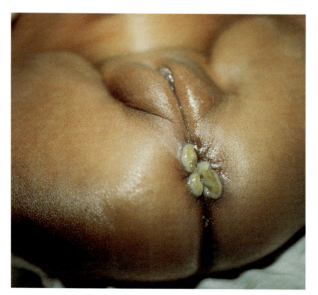

Figure 2.75. Condylomata lata presenting at the age of 6 weeks in an infant with congenital syphilis. The RPR (rapid plasma reagin) was negative at birth but at 6 weeks was reactive with a titer of 1:512. The infant was anemic with a hemoglobin of 4.8 mg/dL, three-plus hematuria, CSF (cerebrospinal fluid) pleocytosis, and a positive CSF VDRL. Lesions responded to penicillin 3 days after treatment was initiated. Condylomata lata appear as flat or raised, moist, wart-like cutaneous lesions, grayish-pink in color. They are smooth, round or oval, and wide-based, often mushroom-like, lesions which may be single or multiple. They occur in moist areas, especially the anogenital regions. They heal without scarring and are highly infectious and must be differentiated from condylomata acuminata which are covered by digitate vegetations.

Figure 2.76. Dactylitis may be a rare finding in congenital syphilis. Note the spindle-shaped appearance of the fingers. This is a rare form of osteochondritis of the small bones of the hands and feet which usually appears between 6 months and 2 years of age. It is commonly found in the metacarpals, proximal phalanges of the hands, and the metatarsals. The swelling gives rise to little pain or discomfort.

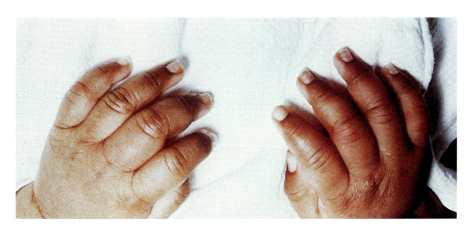

2.76

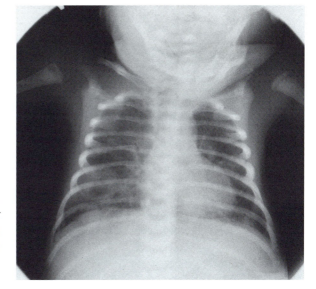

2.77

Figure 2.77. Radiograph of the chest in an infant at age 7 days. The interstitial pneumonia (pneumonia alba) of congenital syphilis is present. This is characterized pathologically by yellowish-white, heavy, firm and grossly enlarged lungs. Note the osseous changes of congenital syphilis at the proximal ends of the humeri.

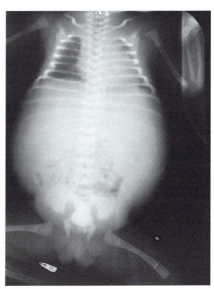

2.78

Figure 2.78. Radiograph of an infant with cogenital syphilis showing massive ascites and growth arrest lines at the ends of long bones.

2.79

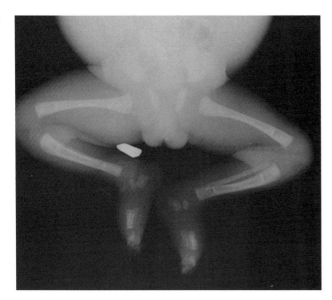

Figure 2.79. This radiograph in the same infant as in Figure 2.78 shows growth arrest lines in the lower extremity long bones. The growth arrest lines at the ends of the long bones are a nonspecific finding in that they signify interference with growth of the fetus in utero and, although commonly seen in congenital syphilis, may occur in many other conditions such as congenital viral infections and erythroblastosis fetalis.

2.80

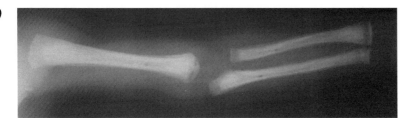

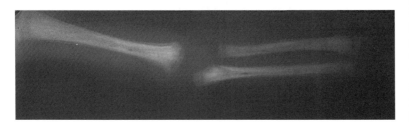

Figure 2.80. Growth arrest lines found in the upper extremities in an infant with congenital syphilis. Growth arrest lines show an enhanced zone of provisional calcification (radiopaque band) which is associated with osteoporosis immediately below the dense zone. The growth arrest line may be smooth or serrated. A serrated appearance is known as Wegner's sign.

Figure 2.81. Radiograph of the upper extremity of an infant with congenital syphilis showing growth arrest lines, periostitis, and fracture of the ulna. Periostitis is seldom visualized at birth because of lack of sufficient calcification at that time to cast a shadow. It is more commonly seen at 4 to 6 weeks of age and, at that time, must be distinguished from that seen in healing rickets, child abuse, and infantile cortical hyperostosis. As the bone is more fragile with syphilitic infection, bone trauma is more common.

2.81

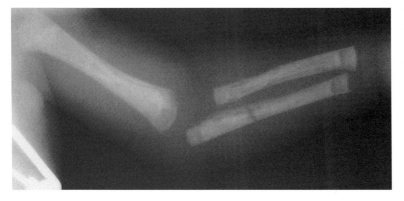

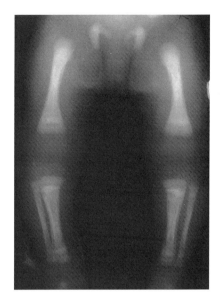

2.82

Figure 2.82. This radiograph demonstrates the lack of ossification centers and the presence of growth arrest lines in the lower extremities of a term infant with congenital syphilis. In congenital syphilis, some growth retardation may occur and it is not unusual to see a delay in appearance of the ossification centers. The bony involvement tends to be multiple and symmetrical. Characteristically bony involvement is widespread and includes the long bones, cranium and ribs. In most cases the osseous lesions are asymptomatic, but in some infants severe involvement may lead to subepiphyseal fractures with epiphyseal dislocation resulting in a painful pseudoparalysis (Parrot's atrophy of newborn). This may mimic Erb's palsy.

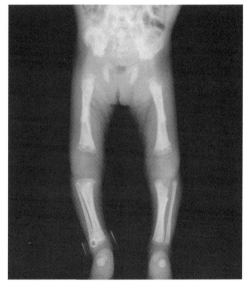

2.83

Figure 2.83. Lower extremity radiograph showing characteristic erosions of syphilitic osteochondritis at the metaphyses of the distal ends of the long bones. About 15% of infants with osteochondritis will show signs at birth. Ninety percent will show radiologic evidence of osteochondritis and periostitis after the first month of life. In osteochondritis, there is increased widening of the epiphyseal lines with increased density of the shafts, spotty areas of radiolucency, and a resultant moth-eaten appearance.

2.84

Figure 2.84. Radiograph of lower extremities and right upper extremity in this infant at the age of 7 days shows the typical syphilitic osteochondritis and some periosteal reaction, especially of the femora. The osteochondritis may be present at birth or may appear during the first month of life. It is most clearly seen in the long bones. The changes seen are fragmentation and apparent destruction with mottled areas of radiolucency.

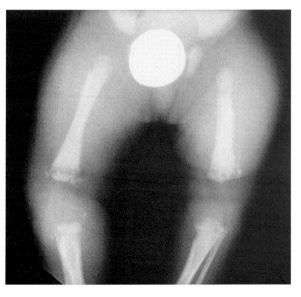
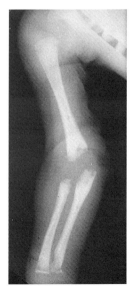

2.85

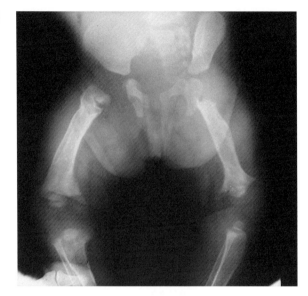

Figure 2.85. Radiograph of the lower extremities of the same infant as in Figure 2.84 at age 6 months. Note the marked alterations of the contour and thickness of the femora. The cortex is thin and the medullary cavity is expanded. The proximal end of the left femur is severely damaged due to syphilitic osteomyelitis. This may present as a syphilitic arthritis of the hip. In spite of these extensive changes, infantile luetic osteitis usually improves remarkably.

2.86

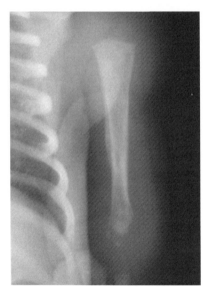

Figure 2.86. Radiograph of the left humerus in an infant with congenital syphilis showing periostitis which was present at birth. The lesions of periostitis are usually diffuse and frequently extend over the entire length of the involved bone. It is first seen as a thin even line of calcification outside the cortex of the involved bone; the lesions progress and eventually produce calcification and thickening of the cortex. When severe, this leads to a permanent deformity such as anterior bowing of the tibia (saber shins). Periostitis of the frontal bones of the skull, when severe, is responsible for the flat overhanging forehead that may persist as a stigma of congenital syphilis in infancy.

2.87

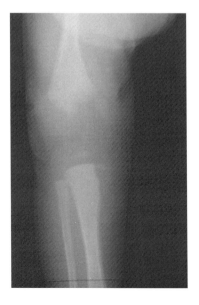 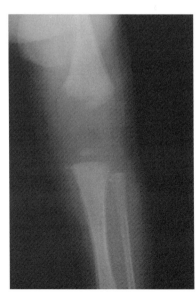

Figure 2.87. Wimberger's sign in an infant with congenital syphilis is recognized by radiolucency due to erosion of the medial aspect of the proximal tibial metaphysis. Painless effusion in one or both knees (Clutton's joints) generally becomes apparent between 8 to 15 years of age, involutes spontaneously and leaves no residual effects.

2.88

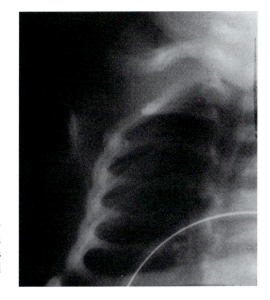

Figure 2.88. Higouménaki's sign refers to periostitis of the clavicle. This may be observed clinically or radiographically and is a diagnostic finding in congenital syphilis. Note also the periostitis of the ribs. Fracture of the clavicle with callus formation should be a consideration in the differential diagnosis.

VIRAL INFECTION

2.89

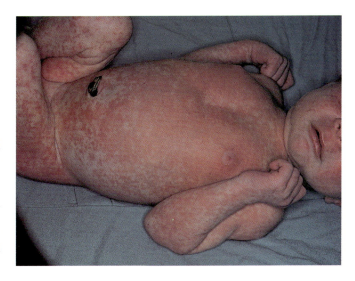

Figure 2.89. This infant at age 5 days developed fever, lethargy and poor feeding. On sepsis evaluation there was a pleocytosis of 120 WBCs in the cerebrospinal fluid indicative of meningoencephalitis. There was no evidence of cardiac involvement. The following day the infant developed a generalized maculopapular rash and loose stools. He recovered without treatment. Stool culture grew Coxsackie virus.

2.90

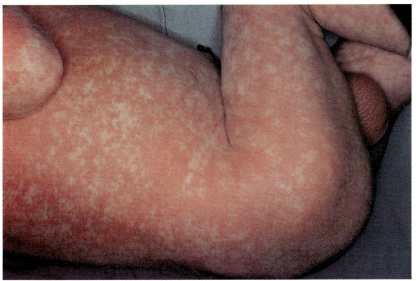

Figure 2.90. Close-up view of the rash from the same infant as in Figure 2.89 with Coxsackie virus infection.

2.91

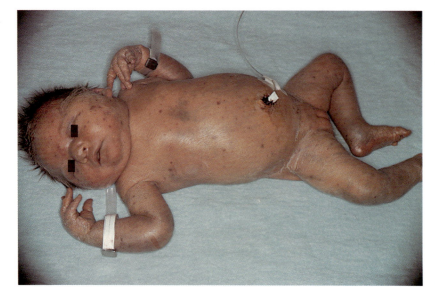

Figure 2.91. This infant with cytomegalovirus infection has a low birthweight due to intrauterine growth retardation and shows the "blueberry muffin" appearance, microcephaly, and abdominal distention due to marked hepatosplenomegaly. Cytomegalovirus infection is asymptomatic in approximately 90% of infected infants at birth. Of these, 5 to 10% develop late-onset sequelae such as hearing loss, chorioretinitis, mental retardation, and neurologic sequelae. The remaining 10% may have mild to severe and occasionally fatal disease.

2.92

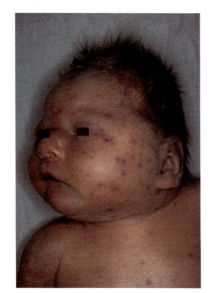

Figure 2.92. A close-up of the head and face of the same infant as in Figure 2.91 with microcephaly and the typical "blueberry muffin" lesions. These lesions represent areas of dermal erythropoiesis. Cutaneous manifestations include petechiae, purpura, "blueberry muffin" lesions (also seen in congenital rubella and other conditions), and vasculitis.

2.93

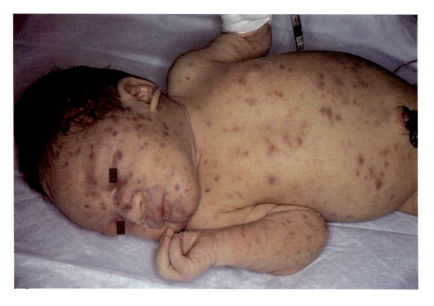

Figure 2.93. Another infant with cytomegalovirus infection showing the typical "blueberry muffin" appearance and jaundice soon after birth. Note that the head size is normal. Since most infections are asymptomatic, early diagnosis is only made in the full-blown syndrome manifested by the appearance of jaundice within the first 24 hours of life, hepatosplenomegaly, abdominal distention, anemia, thrombocytopenia, respiratory distress and neurologic changes.

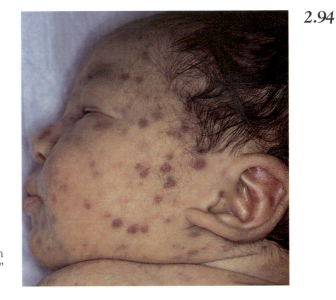

2.94

Figure 2.94. Close-up of the face of the same infant as in Figure 2.93 showing the typical "blueberry muffin" appearance.

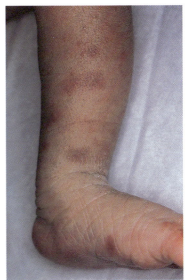

2.95

Figure 2.95. This infant presented with areas of skin involvement on the extremities only. The lesions were asymmetrical in that they were present on the right leg and left arm. Vasculitis, a less common manifestation of skin involvement by cytomegalovirus infection, was confirmed by skin biopsy.

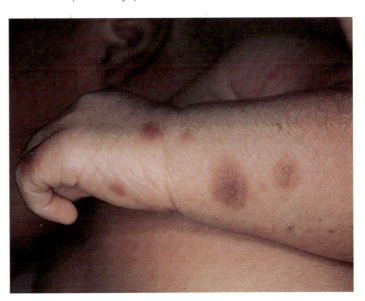

2.96

Figure 2.96. Lesions on the left arm of the same infant as in Figure 2.95 show the vasculitis.

2.97

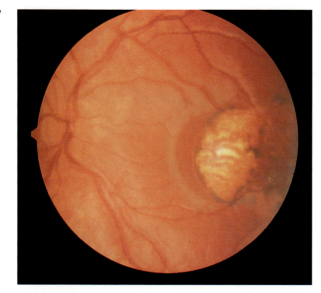

Figure 2.97. Macular chorioretinitis which is typical of cytomegalovirus infection.

2.98

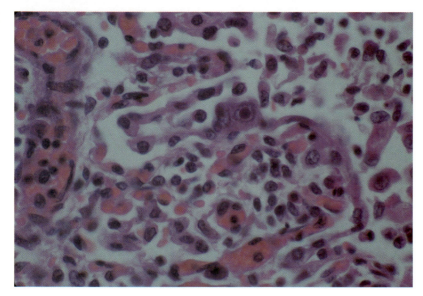

Figure 2.98. Histopathologic section of lung demonstrating the typical "owl's eye" appearance of cells infected with cytomegalovirus. Postnatally acquired cytomegalovirus infection can occur in infants with primary immunodeficiencies or following transfusion with cytomegalovirus-positive blood, etc. (Langston, C.)

2.99

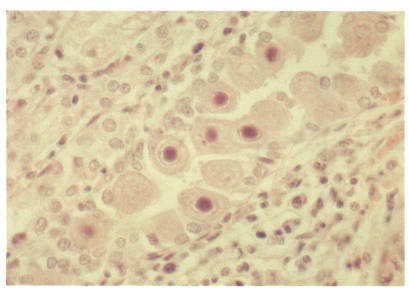

Figure 2.99. "Owl's eye" appearance in a histopathologic section of the kidney. Note the large cellular size which results from an increase in volume of both the nucleus and the cytoplasm. The nuclear inclusion is located centrally and corresponds to the shape of the cell. The nucleolus is usually displaced peripherally in infected cells. There is no necrosis of cells. (Langston, C.)

2.100

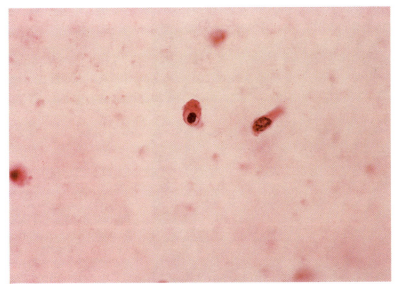

Figure 2.100. Typical "owl's eye" cells in the urine in an infant infected with cytomegalovirus. These cells are distinctive and large, containing intranuclear and cytoplasmic inclusions. (Langston, C.)

2.101

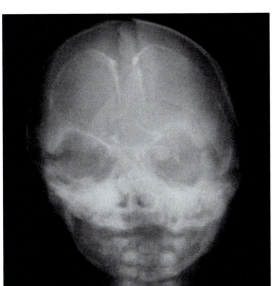

Figure 2.101. Radiograph showing the postero-anterior view of the skull of an infant infected with cytomegalovirus. Note the severe microcephaly and periventricular calcifications. These calcifications demonstrate the marked enlargement of both lateral ventricles. The changes were present at birth.

2.102

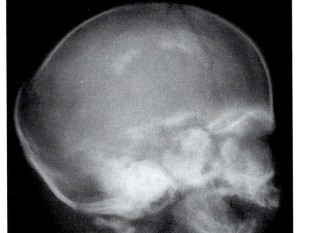

Figure 2.102. Lateral radiograph of the skull of the same infant as in Figure 2.101, again demonstrating microcephaly and periventricular calcifications. Periventricular calcification is seen most commonly in congenital cytomegalovirus infection whereas intracranial calcification in congenital toxoplasmosis is usually more generalized.

2.103

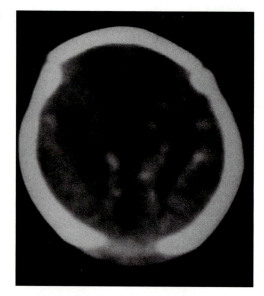

Figure 2.103. CT scan of the head shows periventricular calcifications and dilatation of the ventricles in an infant infected with cytomegalovirus. Intracranial calcification is present in about 20% of infected infants and may be noted much earlier on CT than on initial skull radiographs.

2.104

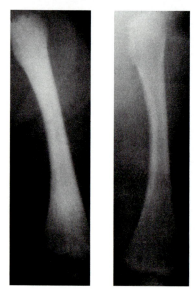

Figure 2.104. The radiograph on the left shows the typical "celery stalk" appearance at the distal end of the femur. This appearance is commonly found in infants with congenital rubella, but on rare occasions can be seen in infants infected with cytomegalovirus. The radiograph on the right shows resolution of the abnormal findings at 1 month of age.

2.105

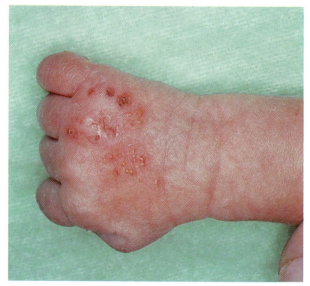

Figure 2.105. Herpetic lesions which appeared on the hand of an infant at the age of 5 days. The skin only was involved in this infant. There was rapid improvement on treatment with intravenous acyclovir. Infection may be acquired as the fetus passes through the birth canal. Thus, although skin lesions may be present at birth, the clinical picture of herpes in the newborn is frequently that of an apparently well infant who becomes symptomatic on the 4th to 8th day of life. The spectrum of illness in herpes simplex virus infection is broad ranging, from death or recovery with severe central nervous system or ocular damage to mild or asymptomatic infection with apparent complete recovery.

2.106

Figure 2.106. Herpetic lesions which appeared on the skin at 7 days of age in an infant who developed disseminated herpes simplex. Herpetic skin lesions are confluent, fluid-filled vesicles with an erythematous halo around the base. These vesicles become pustular after 24 to 48 hours and eventually become crusted or ulcerated. Most neonatal herpes simplex virus infections (80%) are caused by Type II (genital) herpes virus, acquired either by ascending infection from the mother's genital area to the fetus or by spread during delivery through the birth canal of the infected mother. Infection may be acquired by transplacental spread (about 5% of cases) or by postnatal contact with other infants or personnel with oral herpes simplex virus infections.

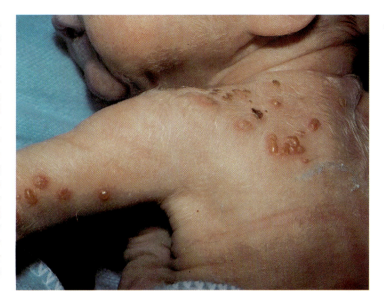

2.107

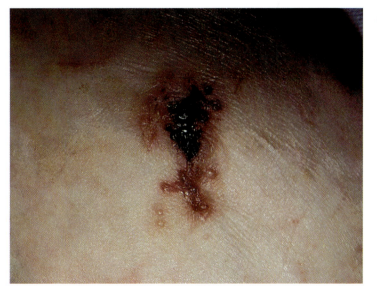

Figure 2.107. The same infant as in Figure 2.106 developed a fresh crop of skin lesions in the periumbilical area five days later while on systemic therapy. This is not uncommon as herpetic lesions often appear in crops. This infant also had herpes simplex encephalitis. Seventy percent of infants with neonatal herpes simplex virus infection have skin lesions, and 70% of these, if left untreated, will progress to systemic infection. Therefore, treat early.

2.108

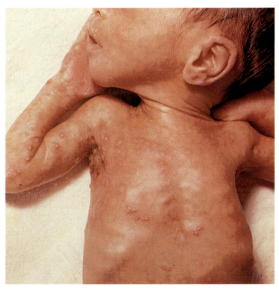

Figure 2.108. Disseminated neonatal herpes simplex infection in a premature infant who presented with skin involvement at age 6 days. The eruption is zosteriform and has been described in infants with herpes simplex virus infection. Skin lesions that may occur include petechiae, purpura, zosteriform lesions, erythematous macular lesions that eventually develop vesicles within the macules, pustular erosions, and large bullae. About 80% of infected babies develop skin lesions between 1 and 4 weeks of age.

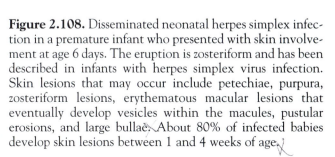

2.109

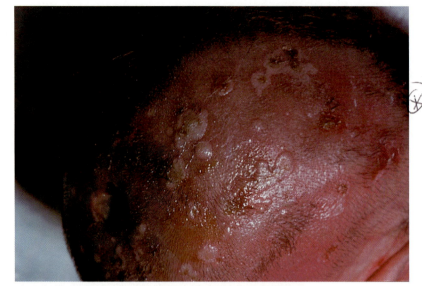

Figure 2.109. Herpetic skin lesions on the scalp in a premature infant (birthweight 1450 g). These lesions on the scalp appeared at the age of 4 days. Occasionally the presenting part of the infant at delivery may be covered by a diffuse edematous swelling resembling that seen in a caput succedaneum. Rather than resolving during the first week, this may become boggy and necrotic with a resultant draining sinus or eschar formation and tense irregular herpetic vesicles.

2.110

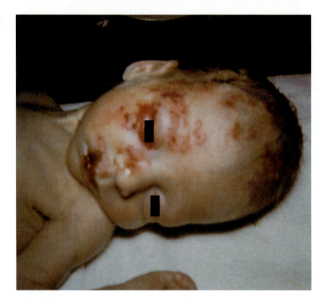

Figure 2.110. Disseminated neonatal herpes simplex infection with skin lesions on the face and eyelids. This infant had keratitis and encephalitis. At times conjunctivitis and keratoconjunctivitis may be seen as the first presenting signs of neonatal herpes infection. This is subsequently followed by lethargy, poor feeding, temperature instability, jaundice, hepatosplenomegaly, and widespread herpes simplex dissemination.

2.111

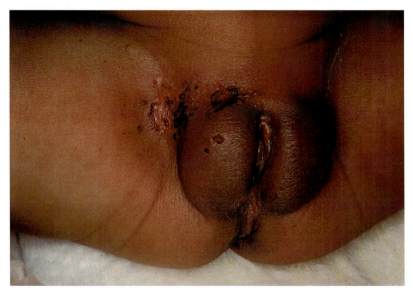

Figure 2.111. Herpetic lesions present on the vulva following a breech presentation. Note also the presence of ecchymoses. Skin lesions occur most often on the scalp and face, the areas which are closest to and in longest contact with the cervical area from which infection is transmitted. Involvement of the cornea in vertex presentations and the genitalia in breech presentations is thus common in herpetic infection.

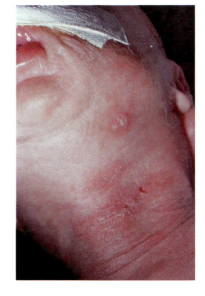

2.112

crxfr the lab

Figure 2.112. Herpetic skin lesions on the neck of a premature infant. A simple Gram stain or Tzanck test would differentiate this from staphylococcal infection. The presence of multinucleated giant cells containing intranuclear inclusions (balloon cells) are characteristic of viral infection.

2.113

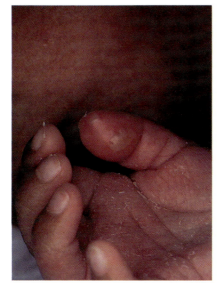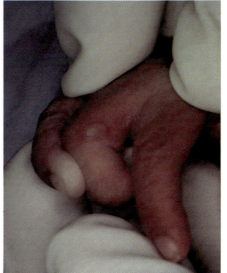

Figure 2.113. This infant with severe intrauterine growth retardation developed herpetic skin lesions and encephalitis. The infant was treated with acyclovir and improved, but the EEG and CT scan were grossly abnormal. One month following treatment he developed a fresh crop of lesions on the right hand (vesicles with paronychia) with resolution after a second course of acyclovir.

2.114

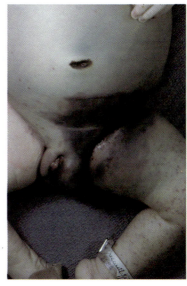

Figure 2.114. This infant presented with cardiovascular collapse and disseminated intravascular coagulopathy. She was well until age 12 days at which time she developed massive ecchymoses and petechiae with bleeding from the umbilical stump and rectum. There was rapid deterioration and death within 2 hours. Autopsy showed disseminated herpetic lesions. There may be hepatitis, pneumonia, coagulopathy with severe bleeding diathesis, and disease of the central nervous system (meningoencephalitis).

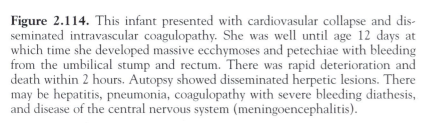

2.115

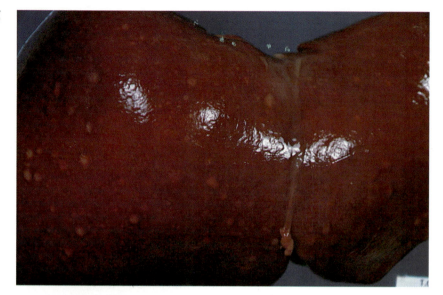

Figure 2.115. Gross pathologic specimen of the liver of the same infant as in Figure 2.114 showing herpetic lesions. The disseminated form of neonatal herpes simplex infection affects the visceral organs, chiefly the liver and adrenal glands. It may also involve the CNS and other organs, and results in a high mortality.

2.116

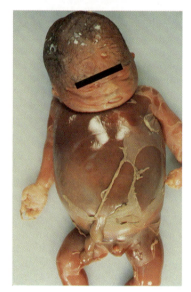

Figure 2.116. Parvovirus B19 infection resulting in intrauterine death in a hydropic stillbirth. Human parvovirus B19, the same virus that causes erythema infectiosum, has a special affinity for rapidly dividing cells, particularly erythroblasts; therefore, an infection may result in profound anemia, hydrops fetalis, and death in the fetus. (Singer, D.)

2.117

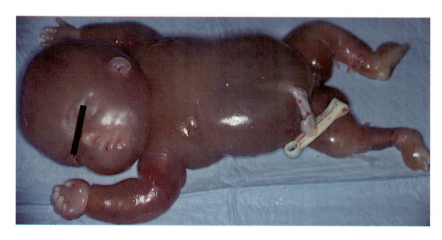

Figure 2.117. Nonimmune hydrops fetalis due to parvovirus B19 infection in a premature infant born at 24 weeks gestation. Note the gross hydrops fetalis. Laboratory analysis was remarkable for a hemoglobin level of 1.4 g/dL, hematocrit of 4%, platelet count of 10,000/mm^3, and WBC count of 6000/mm^3 (which, when corrected for nucleated red blood cells, showed a WBC count of 0).

2.118

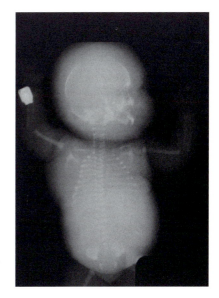

Figure 2.118. Radiograph of the same infant as in Figure 2.117 showing severe hydrops fetalis. Note the massive soft tissue edema. In pregnant women with evidence of infection, maternal serum alphafetoprotein concentration may provide a marker of fetal aplastic crisis. If the concentration is increased, serial ultrasonography may be used to check the possibility of fetal hydrops, and fetal sampling may indicate the severity of fetal anemia. Treatment is by in utero transfusion to the fetus.

2.119

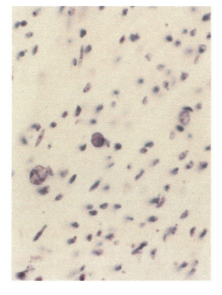 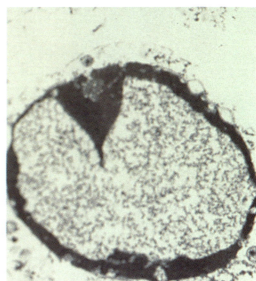

Figure 2.119. Pathologic slide of parvovirus B19 infection in erythroblasts. The virus can be clearly seen on the right in the electron micrograph of a nucleated red cell. (Singer, D.)

2.120

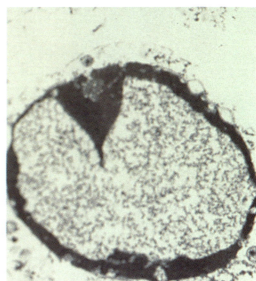

Figure 2.120. Congenital rubella in a term infant with severe intrauterine growth retardation (birthweight 1300 g). Note the "blueberry muffin" appearance. Infected infants are usually born at term, but with low birthweight. In addition to the "blueberry muffin" lesions there may be thrombocytopenic purpura, hyperbilirubinemia, hepatosplenomegaly, pneumonia, congenital cardiac defects (especially patent ductus arteriosus), eye disorders, deafness, and meningoencephalitis.

2.121

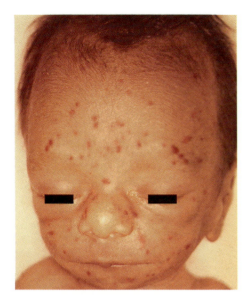

Figure 2.121. Close-up view of the face of the same infant as in Figure 2.120. Note that the "blueberry muffin" lesions in this infant were red rather than purple. In infants with fresh lesions the initial color is dark red but then changes to a bluish-red and dark blue color over the course of a few days. The lesions are infiltrated macules measuring 2 to 8 mm in diameter, are usually present at birth or within the first 24 hours, and new lesions are rare after 2 days.

2.122

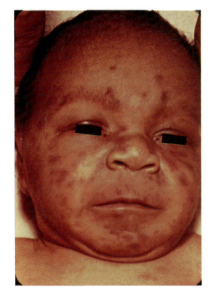

Figure 2.122. This infant shows the typical "blueberry muffin" skin lesions. Histologically, "blueberry muffin" lesions reveal discrete dermal aggregates of relatively large nucleated cells and non-nucleated erythrocytes. They are the result of dermal erythropoiesis (rather than true hemorrhage). These infiltrative lesions, characteristic of viral infections in the fetus, are not unique to infants with congenital rubella but may be seen in congenital cytomegalovirus infection and congenital toxoplasmosis. They also occur in erythroblastosis fetalis, congenital leukemia, etc.

2.123

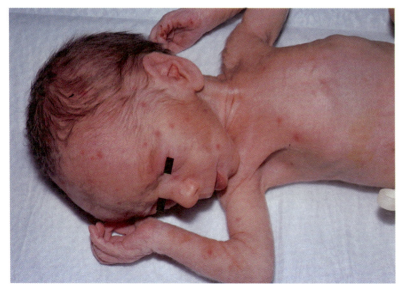

Figure 2.123. The intrauterine growth retardation in congenital rubella may be very striking as shown in this term infant with a birthweight of 860 g. The lesions of congenital rubella may be few or numerous and generally occur on the head, trunk, or extremities. Many of the larger lesions tend to be raised. They usually disappear within 3 to 4 weeks (the larger lesions more slowly than the small flat nodules).

2.124

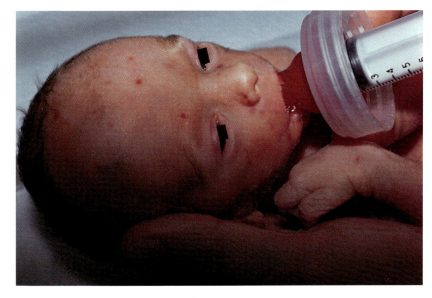

Figure 2.124. Although the infant with congenital rubella was of extremely low birth-weight, he nippled all feeds well. Note the presence of a few "blueberry muffin" lesions.

2.125

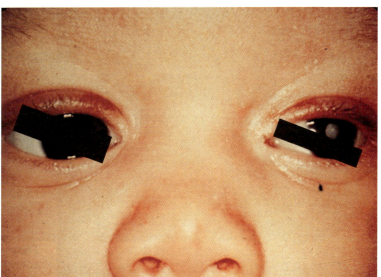

Figure 2.125. Microphthalmia and congenital cataract of the left eye in an infant with congenital rubella.

2.126

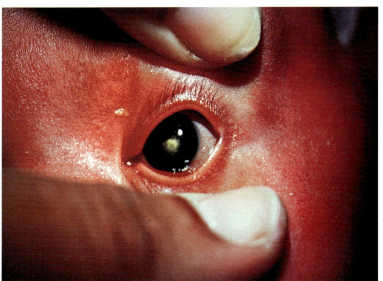

Figure 2.126. Congenital rubella cataract.

2.133

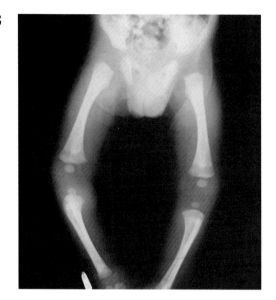

Figure 2.133. Lower extremity radiograph in an infant with congenital rubella at 3 weeks of age. Note the radiolucent zones paralleling the growth plates with residual irregular trabecular pattern. These are the nonspecific growth arrest lines which may be seen in any condition interfering with the growth of the fetus in utero.

2.134

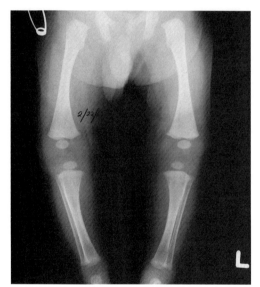

Figure 2.134. Repeat radiographs of the same infant as in Figure 2.133 at 2 months of age showing the regression of these changes.

2.135

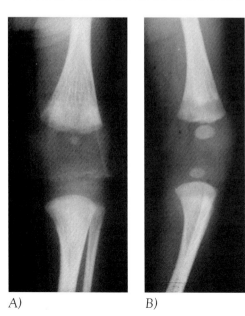

A)   B)   C)

Figure 2.135. Radiograph composite that demonstrates the types of bony changes found in congenital rubella syndrome: from left to right, A) "celery stalk" appearance; B) nonspecific growth arrest lines; C) a bony spicule at the medial condyle of the femur (an uncommon finding). All of these regress over the first few months postnatally.

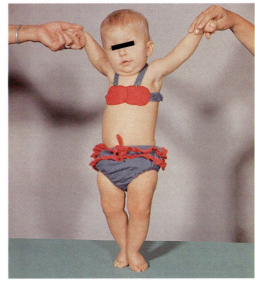

2.136

Figure 2.136. Children with congenital rubella may have a normal physical and neurodevelopmental outcome, although it is uncommon. Maternal rubella in the first 4 weeks of pregnancy carries a risk of congenital rubella of 50% (heart anomalies, eye defects, hearing problems, etc.); between the 12th and 16th weeks of pregnancy the risk decreases to 2 to 6%; and between the 18th to 20th weeks of pregnancy the risk is practically nil. Over 80% of babies with congenital rubella shed virus during the first month of life, and 5 to 10% (those severely affected), for one year.

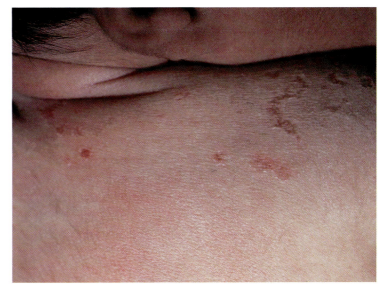

2.137

Figure 2.137. Cicatricial skin lesions of the neck and upper back in an otherwise normal infant following maternal varicella at 5 months gestation. These skin lesions are the most common finding after maternal varicella which presents in the 1st and early 2nd trimester. Maternal infection with varicella early in pregnancy is a cause of fetal malformations including reduction deformities of the limbs (hypoplastic limbs and/or contractures) and scars along the length of the affected limbs. The infant may be small for gestational age and demonstrate features of central nervous system involvement (encephalomyelitis) and eye defects (microphthalmia, cataracts, and chorioretinitis).

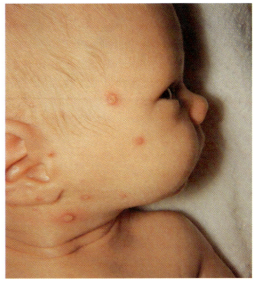

2.138

Figure 2.138. Congenital varicella in an infant which presented at the age of 7 days. Mother developed varicella 10 days prior to delivery. This infant had very few lesions and was not ill. If the onset in the mother is within 4 days prior to or within 48 hours after delivery, or if the onset in the newborn is between 5 to 10 days after birth, the infant's condition is usually more severe. In these cases, varicella-zoster immune globulin (VZIG) should be given as soon as possible after birth.

2.139

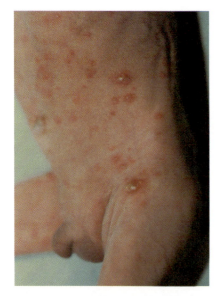 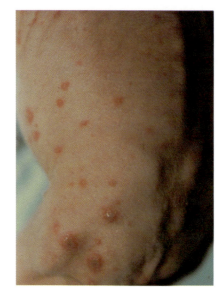

Figure 2.139. Another case of congenital varicella infection. Complications of congenital varicella may be disseminated and fulminant with pneumonia, hepatitis, or encephalomyelitis, and mortality is high. (Cabrera-Meza, G.)

2.140

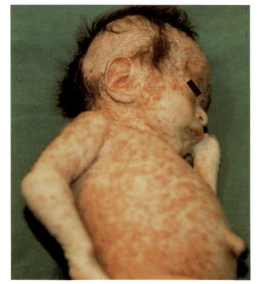

Figure 2.140. This neonate with congenital varicella has extensive skin involvement. (Cabrera-Meza, G.)

2.141

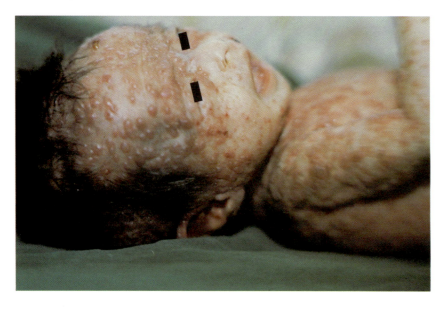

Figure 2.141. Close-up of the same infant as in Figure 2.140 with congenital varicella, showing extensive skin lesions at different stages. (Cabrera-Meza, G.)

PROTOZOAL AND PARASITIC INFECTIONS

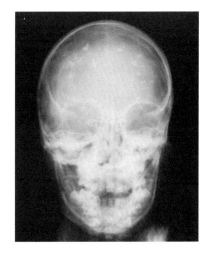

2.142

Figure 2.142. Anteroposterior (AP) skull radiograph in a child with congenital toxoplasmosis. Note the diffuse areas of intracranial calcification. This is characteristic of toxoplasmosis and may be associated subsequently with hydrocephalus or microcephaly. *Toxoplasma gondii* infection is transmitted to the fetus by invasion of the bloodstream during the stage of maternal parasitemia, and may result in a wide spectrum of clinical signs and symptoms. The fetus may be stillborn, born prematurely, or born at full term.

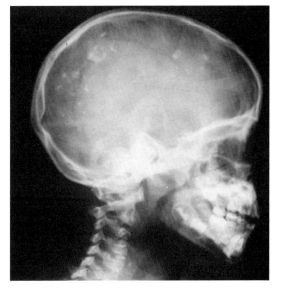

2.143

Figure 2.143. Lateral radiograph from the same child as in Figure 2.142, showing diffuse intracranial calcifications. Intracranial calcifications, in general, are diffuse and scattered in infants with congenital toxoplasmosis. Skull radiographs of infected infants frequently reveal this diffuse punctate intracranial calcification. The distribution of the calcification in infants with congenital cytomegalovirus infection is periventricular.

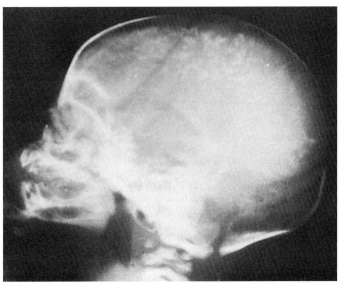

2.144

Figure 2.144. Lateral radiograph of the skull of a newborn infant infected with both toxoplasmosis and cytomegalovirus. Diffuse intracranial calcifications are present.

2.145

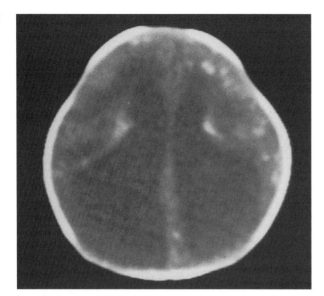

Figure 2.145. A CT scan in an infant with toxoplasmosis at the age of 22 days, showing the scattered intracranial calcification with some brain destruction.

2.146

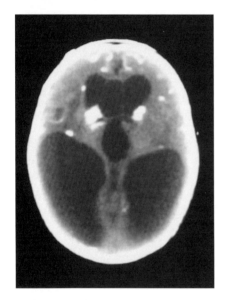

Figure 2.146. The CT scan of another infant at the age of 1 month showed marked brain destruction with scattered intracranial calcifications and hydrocephalus ex vacuo. The illness is usually apparent at birth in that the infant may have fever, poor feeding, vomiting and diarrhea, jaundice, and hepatosplenomegaly. There may be a maculopapular rash or "blueberry muffin" lesions as well as microphthalmia, cataracts, and chorioretinitis. The chorioretinitis is in the region of the macula and is seen in about 80% of infants with congenital toxoplasmosis.

2.147

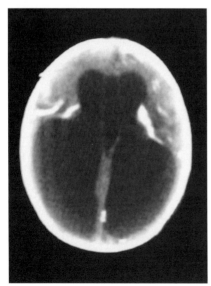

Figure 2.147. CT scan of the same infant several days later with congenital toxoplasmosis. Note the rapid progress with massive loss of brain parenchyma and multiple scattered areas of calcification. Peripheral white blood count was remarkable for 96% eosinophils. There were numerous eosinophils in the cerebrospinal fluid. In toxoplasmosis, anemia, thrombocytopenia, and at times severe leukopenia may be present. The cerebrospinal fluid is xanthochromic, has an elevated protein level, and may contain erythrocytes and leukocytes.

2.148

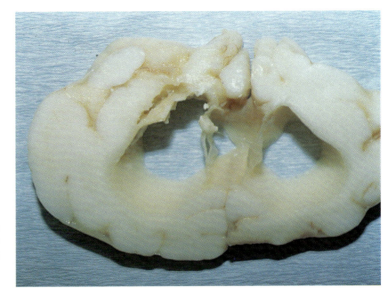

Figure 2.148. Pathologic specimen showing a section of the brain from the same infant as in Figure 2.147. Note the hydrocephalus and cortical necrosis present at autopsy.

2.149

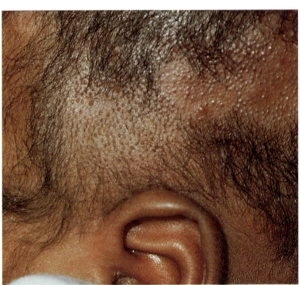

Figure 2.149. This infant has neonatal tinea capitis (ringworm), which was diagnosed at the age of 3 weeks. The condition is rarely seen in the neonate. Lesions are sharply outlined and ring- or disc-shaped, and there may be confluent areas of alopecia with areas of broken and brittle hair observed on an erythematous, scaling scalp (silvery scales). The diagnosis of ringworm of the scalp can frequently be made by the presence of fluorescence under a Wood's light (the affected scalp appears green due to fluorescence of the infected hairs) or by microscopic examination of infected hairs. In the neonate, the infection is usually produced by *Microsporon canis*, *M. audouinii*, or *Trichophyton tonsurans*. The hair does not fluoresce in a *Trychophyton tonsurans* infection. (Levy, M., Moise, K.)

2.150

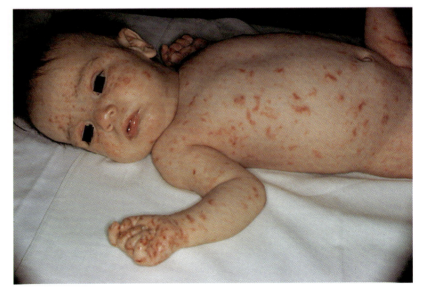

Figure 2.150. This infant presented with scabies at the age of 17 days. The mother had scabies. This parasitic infection is uncommon in the neonate. The distribution of the lesions is different from that of the older child in that the face, head, and neck may be involved, especially if the mother is breastfeeding. There may be scabetic burrows, papules, and vesicular lesions. In addition there is involvement of the usual areas such as the flexor surfaces of the extremities, the interdigital spaces, the groins and the axilla.

2.151

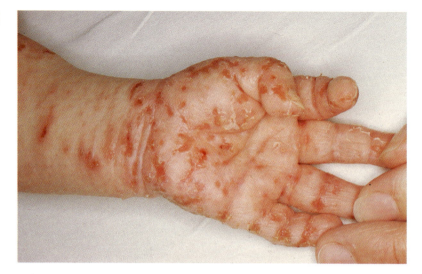

Figure 2.151. A close-up of the hand in the same infant as in Figure 2.150 showing the typical scabetic lesions. Primary lesions are burrows, papules, and vesicular lesions. Secondary bacterial infection causing pustules may occur.

2.152

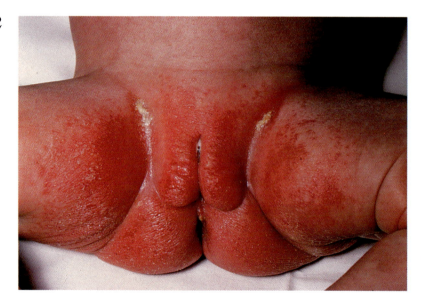

Figure 2.152. Typical candidal diaper dermatitis. Note the symmetric distribution of the rash with involvement of the intertriginous areas. Satellite lesions are often present. The skin is erythematous, swollen and slightly scaly. With healing, areas of depigmentation may occur. This should be differentiated from an ammoniacal diaper dermatitis where the rash is generally asymmetric, the intertriginous areas are spared, and satellite lesions are absent as it is a contact dermatitis.

2.153

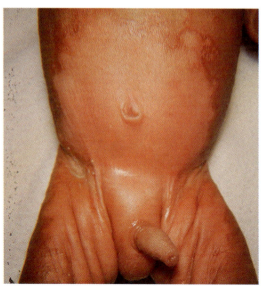

Figure 2.153. An infant with healed candidal dermatitis showing symmetrical depigmentation. Note the healed satellite areas. Candidal (monilial) dermatitis is a commonly overlooked disorder and should be suspected whenever a diaper rash fails to respond to usual measures.

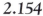

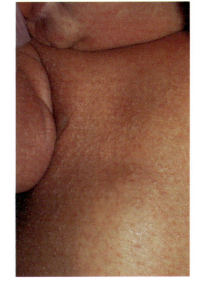

2.154

Figure 2.154. Congenital cutaneous candidiasis in an infant at age 3 days. Potassium hydroxide (KOH) scrapings of the skin were positive for hyphae. Mucocutaneous candidiasis may present as a vesicular dermatitis in the first week of life. The vesicular lesions become confluent and rupture, leaving a denuded area surrounded by satellite lesions or pustules. Congenital candidiasis may have only skin manifestations or there may be severe systemic involvement following the intrauterine infection.

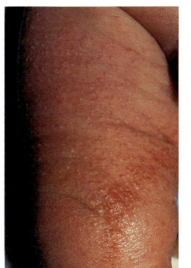

2.155

Figure 2.155. Close-up of the skin of the same infant as in Figure 2.154. Note the pinpoint pustulovesicular lesions. Diagnosis can be confirmed by culture on Sabouraud's or Nickerson's media.

2.156

Figure 2.156. Congenital disseminated mucocutaneous candidiasis in an infant at age 5 days. Note the thrush with the generalized skin rash. These infants are generally well and have no systemic involvement. Although cutaneous candidiasis frequently occurs in association with oral thrush, commonly the mouth is bypassed and the infection is confined exclusively to the diaper area. Infants harbor *Candida albicans* in the lower intestine, and it is from this focus that infected feces present the primary source for candidal diaper rash.

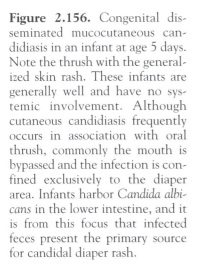

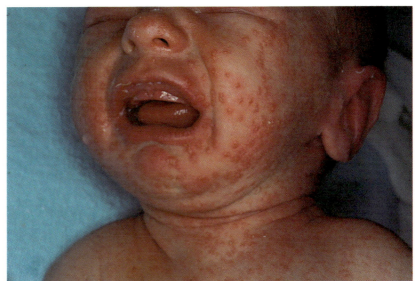

2.157

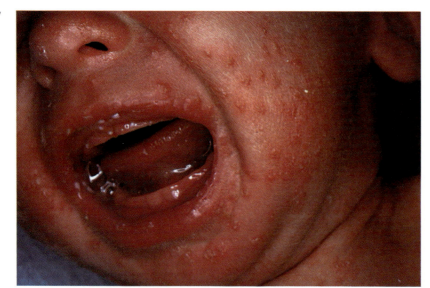

Figure 2.157. Close-up of the mouth and face in the same infant as in Figure 2.156. The white plaques on the tongue and buccal mucosa resemble milk curds; they are difficult to detach from the mucosa and leave a raw erythematous base.

2.158

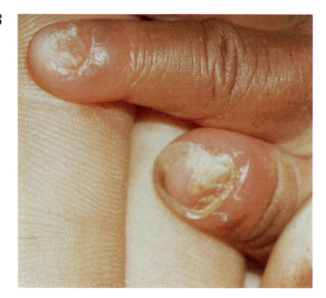

Figure 2.158. This premature infant developed candidal infection of the nails (onychomycosis) at the age of 3 weeks. Premature infants with thrush are more likely to develop infection of the nails from hand-mouth contact. Candidal infection almost exclusively affects the fingernails, whereas tineal infection more frequently affects toenails. In candidal infection the nail plate may be fragile and thick and may show grayish-white spots or brown discoloration of the nail edge. As there frequently is an associated paronychia in candidal infection, the adjacent cuticle is pink, swollen, and tender (caused by secondary staphyloccal infection). (Levy, M., Moise, K.)

2.159

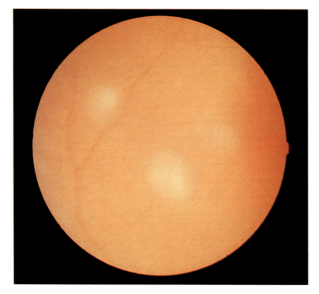

Figure 2.159. Candidal endophthalmitis as represented by the appearance of "cotton" patches is observed in an infant with systemic candidiasis. These lesions are diagnostic of a systemic candidal infection.

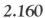

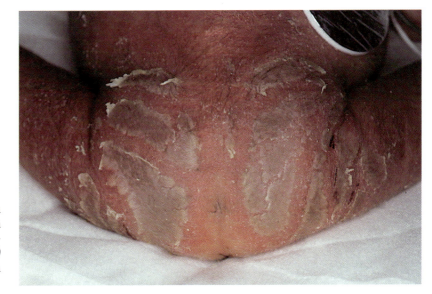

2.160

Figure 2.160. Candidal infection of the back and buttocks in a small premature infant (birthweight 775 g) at the age of 10 days. Hyphae were present both on the skin and in the urine.

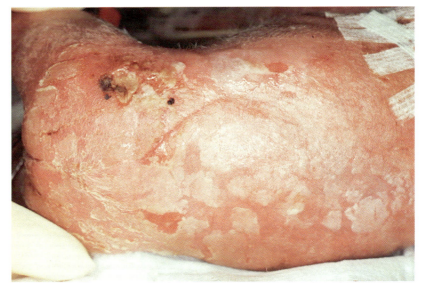

2.161

Figure 2.161. Candidal infection of the back in a premature infant of 24 weeks gestation (birthweight 680 g). The severe skin involvement was noted at 9 days of age when the condition of the infant was stable. There was minimal handling of the infant prior to this. This infant developed a patent ductus arteriosus which required ligation. Intravenous therapy with amphotericin was not successful.

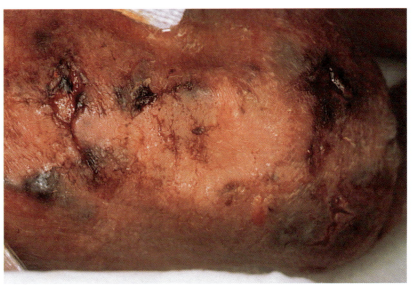

2.162

Figure 2.162. Severe disseminated candidiasis in a premature infant (birthweight 690 g). On the 13th day of life he developed the severe rash on his back. Hyphae were present in these lesions. The infant had resolution of fungemia and skin involvement with amphotericin therapy.

2.163

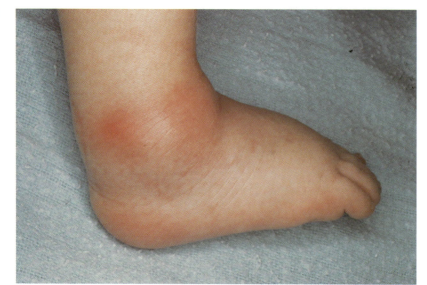

Figure 2.163. Candidal arthritis of the right ankle in an infant who developed candidal sepsis while on prolonged total parenteral nutrition for short bowel syndrome.

2.164

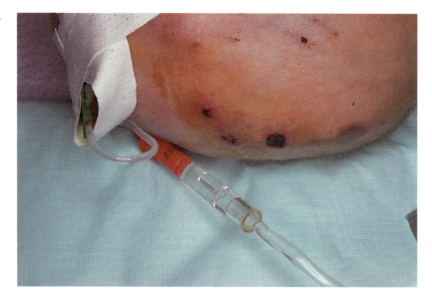

Figure 2.164. Candidal scalp infection in an infant on peripheral parenteral nutrition. The abscesses were recurrent until the cloudy appearance of the infusion solution was noted. Hyphae were seen on examinaton of this fluid. The abscesses resolved with discontinuation of the concentrated glucose solution.

2.165

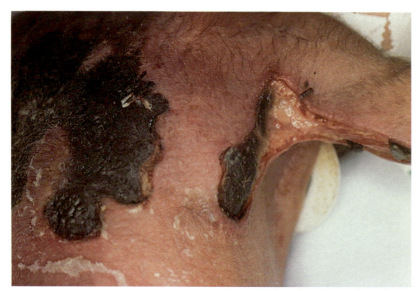

Figure 2.165. Invasive aspergillosis of the skin in a small premature infant (birthweight 785 g) at the age of 7 days. Note the involvement of the back and the right axilla. Infant was treated with amphotericin.

2.166

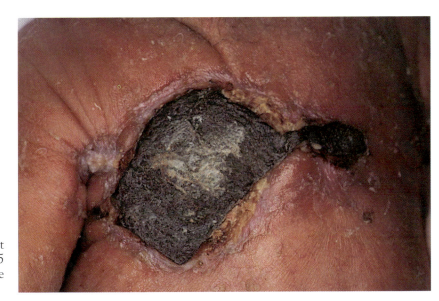

Figure 2.166. The same infant as in Figure 2.165 at the age of 5 weeks, showing healing of the lesions.

2.167

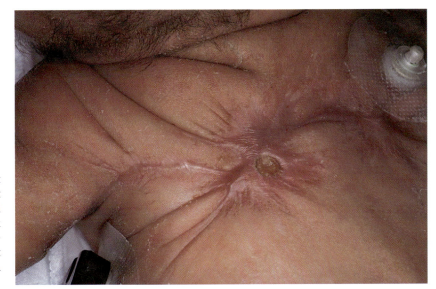

Figure 2.167. The same infant as in Figure 2.165 and 2.166 at the age of 10 weeks with good healing of the skin of the back and axilla. However, the contractures that were present necessitated plastic surgery at a later date.

2.168

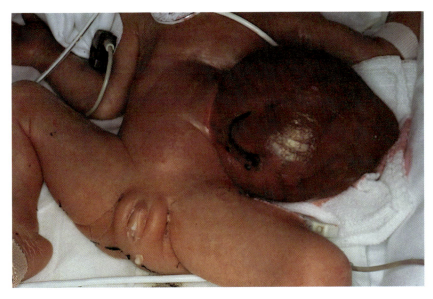

Figure 2.168. Premature infant (birthweight 1000 g) with severe hyaline membrane disease with giant omphalocele. Respiratory problems precluded surgical intervention. The omphalocele was managed medically with the application of mercurochrome. The infant developed mercury intoxication from excessive absorption of the mercurochrome.

2.169

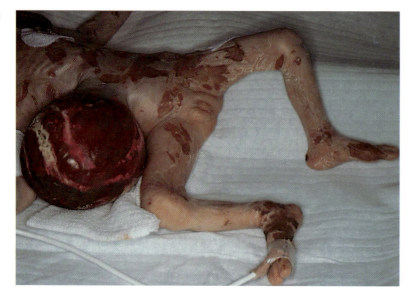

Figure 2.169. The same infant as in Figure 2.168 at the age of 11 days. Note the fungus on the omphalocele. KOH scrapings were positive for hyphae, and culture grew *Aspergillus fumigatus*. Aspergillosis is an uncommon opportunistic fungal disease. *Aspergillus fumigatus* is the most common, but the incidence of *Aspergillus niger* and other species is increasing. These fungi are ubiquitous and normally nonpathogenic. Primarily they affect debilitated individuals.

2.170

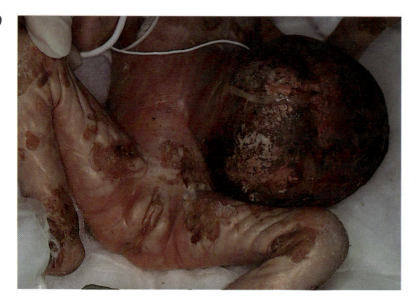

Figure 2.170. The same infant as in Figure 2.168 and 2.169 at the age of 18 days showing generalized involvement of the skin. The skin lesions are characterized by erythematous papules which develop into hemorrhagic bullae and then become violaceous plaques with central necrosis.

2.171

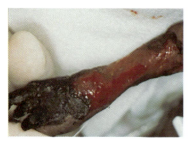

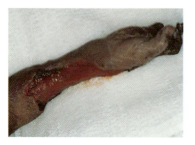

Figure 2.171. This small premature infant born at 23 weeks gestation (birthweight of 580 g) had severe hyaline membrane disease and a large ductus arteriosus. She was referred at the age of 33 days, having developed a *Staphylococcus epidermidis* bacteremia, bilateral grade III intraventricular hemorrhages, and bronchopulmonary dysplasia. Shortly after admission, infection of the right forearm and hand developed which was progressive, becoming gangrenous. *Rhizopus* infection was shown to be the etiology. She died at the age of 83 days.

2.172

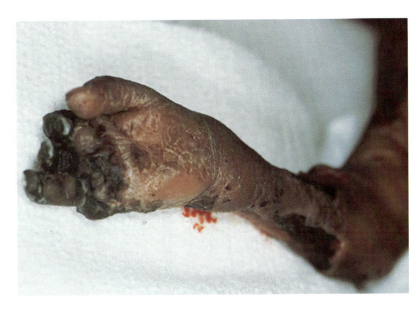

Figure 2.172. Another view of the arm and hand of the same infant as in Figure 2.171. Phycomycosis is very rare in neonates. The most common genera include *Mucor, Absidia,* and *Rhizopus.* Fungi of this class are frequently found in refrigerators and are commonly known as bread molds. Phycomycetes have the same affinity for vascular invasion, hemorrhage, necrosis, and suppuration as *Aspergillus.* There are few reports in the neonatal period, and the majority of these infants have died.

Index